Aphrodisiacs

An Owner's Manual

Aphrodisiacs

An Owner's Manual

Edward Vernon

Illustrated by
John Cameron

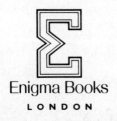

Enigma Books

L O N D O N

British Library Cataloguing in Publication Data

Vernon, Edward
  Aphrodisiacs.
  1. Sex – Anecdotes, facetiae, satire etc.
  I. Title
  306.7′0207   HQ23
  ISBN 0 7278-3004-X

First published in Great Britain in 1982 by
Enigma Books, an imprint of Severn House Publishers
Limited, 4 Brook Street, London W1Y 1AA.

Typeset by Rowland Phototypesetting Limited
Bury St Edmunds, Suffolk.

Printed in Great Britain by Anchor Press Ltd
and bound by Wm. Brendon & Son Ltd,
both of Tiptree, Essex.

CONTENTS

WARNING

The author and publishers wish to make it clear that they are not prepared to accept legal responsibility for any consequences which may be attributed to material contained in this book. Under no circumstances will the author or publishers accept legal liability for pregnancy, marriage, divorce, loss of health, loss of virginity or death from excitement, over stimulation or poisoning.

In addition, we ought to own up, come clean and (not to put too fine a point on it) confess that the names, places and events described in this book are fictitious, imaginary and spurious. What's more, the characters depicted are intended to bear no resemblance whatsoever to persons alive, dead or in limbo.

FOREWORD
by Professor Howard B. Johnstone
Institute of Sexual Chemistry, Maryland, U.S.A.

Much nonsense has been written about aphrodisiacs in recent years. Many myths and legends have been built up for which there is no scientific evidence whatsoever. Ask the average man or woman to name a favourite aphrodisiac and you will probably hear nonsense about substances such as powdered rhinoceros horn or Vitamin E. The real truth is that there is no unequivocal evidence to prove that either of these have any effect at all on sexual desire or frequency. My own Institute knows of no solid scientific work to support the theory that rhinoceros horn is a sexual stimulant and Vitamin E has earned its reputation as an aphrodisiac solely on the basis of a limited amount of research work done on rat fertility patterns.

I believe that one of the reasons why there is so much confusion about aphrodisiacs is that up until now there has never been a comprehensive and reliable guide to this important branch of sexual chemistry. In the absence of solid, easily available information it is easy to make unsubstantiated and misleading claims.

I sincerely hope that, in the future, the science of sexual chemistry will be recognised as a significant branch of clinical pharmacology. The news that a Nobel prize in Sexual Chemistry will be awarded in 1988 must be welcomed by all those working in this delicate area. I would like to see all aphrodisiacs tested accurately and critically and I look forward to the day when objective tests and trials are used to measure sexual endeavour both qualitatively and quantitatively. With this end in sight, my own department is already preparing a list of public-spirited volunteers prepared to put themselves in our hands for the sake of science.

Meanwhile, I wholeheartedly welcome Dr Edward Vernon's majestic contribution to the subject. I believe that it is an accurate and important introduction and I recommend it to all those who have any interest in this fertile field.

Howard B. Johnstone.

AN INTRODUCTORY DEFINITION

The word 'aphrodisiac' is most often used to describe substances which increase libido or sexual desire. It is also frequently used to describe anything that affects sexual performance and is also taken to apply to preparations which improve the quality or quantity of orgasmic experience.

Obviously this single, general, term is likely to cause confusion, so scientists working with Professor Johnstone at the Institute of Sexual Chemistry have divided these different qualities into separate categories. As is often the case with scientists the words they use may seem rather dull and unadventurous. However, I have borrowed their subdivisions to help differentiate between the effects of different substances and I would like to thank Professor Johnstone and his colleagues for permission to reproduce the definitions devised by his Institute.

1. Genital Operant
Any substance which provokes sexual interest and helps to produce discernible results has been dubbed a Genital Operant (G.O.). Occasionally professionals working in this field will refer to G.O.s which affect males only as 'erectants', and those affecting only women as 'moisturizers'.

2. Sexual Trigger and Response Tightener
If, in addition to producing sexual interest, an aphrodisiac encourages sexual action then it is said to have S.T.A.R.T. properties.

3. Performance-lengthening, Ecstasy-amplifying, Sexual Energizer
Any chemical or drug which improves the quality of male or female sexual performance. (P.L.E.A.S.E. is the acronym here).

4. Sexual Inhibition Nullifier
A substance which increases the male sexual repertoire is said to be a Sexual Inhibition Nullifier. A missionary who, thanks to therapeutic intervention, discovers other positions, might be

said to have been disinhibited or converted by a Sexual Inhibition Nullifier. These aphrodisiacs are said to produce the S.I.N. effect.

5. Moment of Response Extender

An aphrodisiac which increases the duration of the peak male or female sexual experience is known as a Moment Of Response Extender (M.O.R.E.).

6. Sensation Quality Unifier, Excacerbator and Lengthener

When an aphrodisiac increases the intensity of an orgasm, it is known as a Sensation Quality Unifier, Excacerbator and Lengthener (S.Q.U.E.A.L.). Because of a secondary effect associated with their use, substances in the category are sometimes known as 'nailbreakers'. Since nailbreaking is often associated with backscratching, married men are usually wise to avoid giving their mistresses aphrodisiacs with S.Q.U.E.A.L. qualities.

PERUVIAN MAGIC
Pheromones

Source and preparation

Sexual interest and activity are stimulated by volatile fatty acids known as pheromones.

These chemical substances are produced naturally by both men and women and it is the quantity and quality of pheromones produced by any individual which determines the style and strength of his or her sexual attraction. A man who finds himself sexually aroused by a young girl is, in fact, attracted by an automatic reflex response to unseen pheromones. He may find specific physical characteristics pleasing, but it is the pheromones which excite him.

Since it is known that the fall in pheromone production which accompanies the ageing process is directly responsible for the accompanying reduction in sexual fortunes, a number of attempts have been made to market pheromones. Moderately successful campaigns involved male pheromones as a component of after shave lotions; but the only completely successful pheromones marketing programme made use of the female pheromone *beta oestradiol* which can, if the correct technique is applied, be obtained from nubile girls.

Known to those who use it as Peruvian Magic ('Peruvian' for reasons that will become apparent later) beta oestradiol is usually sold as a liquid concentrate. In this form it is dabbed onto the pulse points in much the same way as ordinary perfume. It is, however, also possible to have a pheromone implant. The advantage with an implant is that it produces a continuous (albeit slowly decreasing) effect for four to six weeks.

The pheromone concentrate is available only from a retailer in Craven Hill, London. The implants are available from selected gynaecologists.

Type of effect

Pheromones are basically G.O. and S.T.A.R.T. stimulants. They can have a moisturizing effect on some females, particularly tennis players. Pheromones normally act within a range of 15 to 20 feet. Since there is no overt smell with a pheromone, men with mistresses in the older age-range often favour this type of subtle aphrodisiac if they also have suspicious wives.

Speed and length of action
Pheromones begin to work a few seconds after they have been applied to the skin. An implant begins to work instantly (for this reason gynaecologists inserting implants always wear surgical masks). Pheromones applied externally last for six to eight hours. After that time they begin to break down into more primitive chemical constituents which are, in many aspects, indistinguishable from canine pheromones – a fact which can lead to quite considerable embarrassment under certain circumstances.

Warning
The main drawback with pheromones is that they have an effect on all males who come within range. Research done by a German Sexusociology Department has shown that women complaining of sexual harassment at their places of work often produce very high levels of natural pheromones. It is important to remember that pheromones applied externally continue to have a sexually stimulating effect on nearby males whether or not the wearer herself is sexually stimulated.

The use of female pheromones by males is illegal in seventeen American States.

The mystery of Ethel Mitchell
Before I settled down in general practice I worked for a few months as an assistant to an elderly family doctor who had a surgery in the Paddington area of London. While there I lived in a small apartment in an old Victorian house just off Praed Street.

The only problem with the apartment was that it was directly beneath a set of rooms which (according to a small, handwritten piece of white card taped below the appropriate door bell) belonged to a Miss Ethel Mitchell, whose healthy sexual appetite kept me awake hour after hour each night. If you've ever tried to sleep while the bedsprings and floorboards above you are twanging, creaking and vibrating you'll know just what I mean.

I became aware of Miss Mitchell's astonishing appetite as soon as I moved into the apartment; and often, as I set off for the surgery in the morning, I'd meet a young man coming down the stairs from her rooms. It was always a different lover; but each

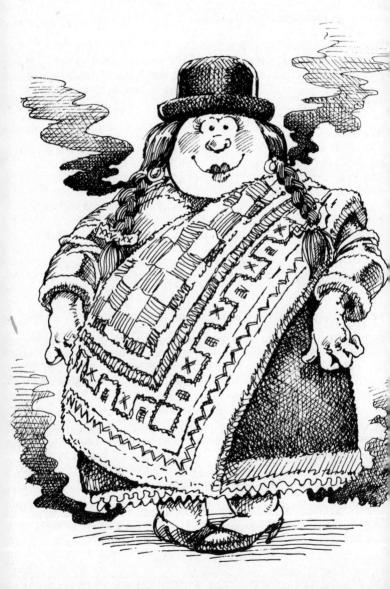

one struggled down with much the same look of contentment and exhaustion as his predecessor. But although I knew something of her tastes and had encountered a number of her boyfriends I hadn't seen Miss Mitchell herself.

As the weeks went by, my curiosity grew. I took to hanging about on the landing, hoping to catch a glimpse of the elusive and mysterious Miss Mitchell. I'd stand around for half an hour at a time pretending to repair the frayed edge of the stair carpet.

When I finally managed to meet her, I was so startled that I fear my surprise showed. Given the vigour and frequency of the action upstairs, I'd thought of Miss Mitchell as being a young and extraordinarily attractive creature. Far from it. She was in her mid-fifties, a little over five feet tall, slight, rather pale and somewhat gloomy looking. Her figure was shapeless and her hair was grey and quite straight. She wore a very old fashioned black coat, a small grey hat with a couple of feathers in it and a pair of sensible low-heeled black shoes. She had bad arthritis in her hands and wore a hearing aid behind her right ear. And yet . . . when I met her I felt a strange and quite inexplicable stirring in my loins. It was the sort of below-the-belt glow that I'd learnt to associate with much younger, much more attractive members of her sex.

Puzzled, bewildered, aroused and extremely curious, I decided to try and find out more about this extraordinary person. After all, it isn't often that you come across little old ladies with enough vigour and style to send an apparently unending series of lovers limping happily down the stairs and enough sex appeal to keep a second series striding expectantly upwards.

For several days I followed Miss Mitchell every time she left her apartment and eventually discovered that the only oddity in her behaviour was that she regularly visited a literary agency in Craven Hill, just around the corner from where we both lived. Clearly, she didn't work there; she never stayed for more than a few minutes; and I found it difficult to believe that a writing career could justify such frequent visits. I decided that there had to be some link between these visits and Miss Mitchell's unusual sexual appeal.

It took three visits to the agency, and a lot more snooping beside before I found the evidence I was seeking. To my astonishment I discovered that the literary agency was a front for a cleverly-disguised organisation offering the world's first commercial trade in pheromones.

For twenty years, it seemed, an anthropologist – whom we

had better refer to as Dr Kingman – had been secretly marketing, from the Craven Hill Office, a special perfume made from the intimate secretions of young Peruvian girls. Having realised that the sexual attractiveness usually associated with young girls is less to do with appearance or age than the hormones they secrete, this skilled scientist had found a way to obtain the secretions, distil them and turn them into a perfume that could be sold to women in their fifties, sixties, seventies and even eighties whose own ability to produce such hormones had long since disappeared. During his travels among remote tribespeople, he had discovered (or so the information I bought led me to believe) a tribe in Peru whose young women produced an unusually powerful pheromone. As evidence of this, the male members of the tribe seemed to spend most of their waking hours in a state of intense sexual excitation. Quick to spot a marketable product, Kingman had set to work to (in effect) 'extract' and bottle lust.

Miss Mitchell, I discovered, was just one of many older women who had become regular customers. Instead of spending their money on clothes, cosmetics and plastic surgery they bought sexual attractiveness in a bottle from Craven Hill. What's more, the anthropologist is still in business. If you visit Craven Hill in London, and keep observation for a while, you'll see a steady stream of elderly ladies still visiting the 'literary agency' there.

A LOVELY PEAR
Bromocriptine

Source and preparation

It has been known for some time that the chemical substance bromocriptine increases the sexual drive in men. Only within the last few years, however, have researchers discovered that there is a strong natural source of bromocriptine in the avocado fruit. This natural bromocriptine is normally inactivated by enzymes but Dr Helmut Wegel, who works at a Scandinavian Institute for Applied Toxicology, recently published a paper in the International Journal of Vegetable Toxicology, showing that the inactivating enzyme can be neutralised by a substance called methylenedioxyamphetamine. This chemical, which occurs naturally in nutmeg, is the only major hallucinogenic amphetamine. To put it another way, the polysyllabic stuff in avocado that turns you on is locked up; something with an even longer name sets it free. This liberator of lust is found in nutmeg. Now proceed . . .

Since the methylenedioxyamphetamine in nutmeg takes between twelve and twenty-four hours to inactivate the enzyme which restricts bromocriptine's sexually stimulating action, this recipe for sexual pleasure needs to be prepared a day or so before use.

Simply sprinkle a quarter of an ounce of grated nutmeg onto the surface of an avocado-half and put it into the refrigerator to await its hour.

Type of effect

Methylenedioxyamphetamine itself produces a sense of euphoria and a general sexual awareness. It has a modest G.O. effect on males but not on women. Released bromocriptine has a S.T.A.R.T. effect, and a mild S.I.N. quality for males.

The cumulative effect of these varied powers makes avocado an excellent general aphrodisiac for use by the predatory female.

Speed and length of action

Methylenedioxyamphetamine has an effect within thirty to sixty minutes. The released bromocriptine takes sixty to ninety minutes. This means that when avocado with nutmeg is served as a starter the subsequent courses should be designed for completion within a maximum of ninety minutes.

Nutmeg with avocado is not a suitable restaurant dish unless private rooms are available since the effect of both methylenedioxyamphetamine and bromocriptine wear off within two to three hours.

Warning

Avocado appetizer is one of the safest aphrodisiacs available. It is known, however, that a small proportion of males (reported figures vary between one in fifty and one in two hundred and fifty) will react unpredictably when given a mixture of bromocriptine and methylenedioxyamphetamine. When this happens the disinhibiting effect on the male can be considerable.

In 1979 a 130 pound male bank clerk in Nice, France, who had been given an avocado appetizer, repeatedly sodomized his wife, sister and brother-in-law for nearly eighteen hours.

Avocado is the food of love – eat on!

Joyce Tavistock had been trying to seduce Malcolm Jackson for nearly four months. During that time she'd never managed to get him to do anything more daring than put a hand on her knee; and she'd only got him to do that by persuading him to hold a patch in place while she repaired a tear in her jeans.

She'd tried buying him chocolates and sending him flowers but that hadn't got her any more than a peck on the cheek and a thank-you note delivered by second-class mail. She'd tried dropping her handkerchief on the floor and bending forward to pick it up so that he could get a good view of her cleavage. All he'd done in response to that provocation was suggest that paper tissues would be more hygienic. She'd taken him to the cinema, worn a dress that buttoned all the way down the front and made sure that they sat in the back row. He'd resolutely watched the travelogue, the advertisements and the movie without so much as offering to share his popcorn with her.

She'd even organised an evening with him in the living-room of her flat while the girl she shared the apartment with and her boyfriend punished bedsprings in the room next door. But Malcolm had mistaken the twanging and twinging for the gurglings of a disordered plumbing system and had thoughtfully recommended a neighbourhood plumber.

After all this had been going on for four months, Joyce began

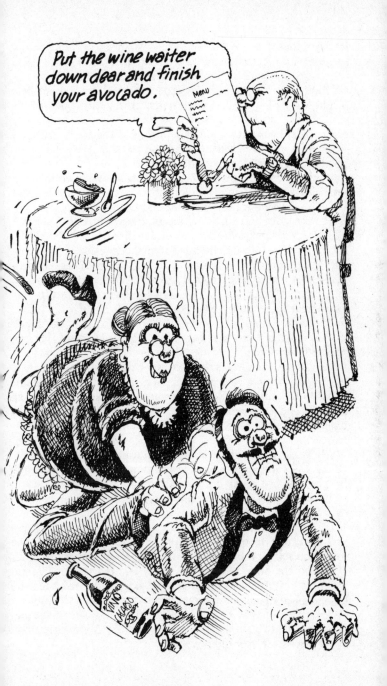

to think that there was something wrong with her. She would never have admitted it to anyone but Malcolm didn't even know that she had a small birthmark on her left breast.

Hope came from a quite unexpected quarter when her best friend Mildred, who had large spots, greasy hair, body-odour and no bust to speak of, came to work with a broad smile, love bites on her neck, a twinkle in her eyes and amazing stories of a weekend spent in Wigan with a bank clerk called Gerald. She also had the recipe for Avocado Appetizer.

Working on the understandable premise that anything that worked for Mildred and Gerald really ought to work for her and Malcolm, Joyce went out the same afternoon and bought a crate full of avocados and six large cans of grated nutmeg. Then she rang Malcolm and invited him round to dinner.

No one could have done more to make an evening a success than Joyce did. She borrowed a dress that would have made a topless waitress appear modest, and sprayed herself with seven different perfumes from the sample bottles in four different local department stores. She bought two litres of fizzy cider, picked off the labels and replaced them with labels she'd cut from champagne advertisements in a glossy magazine. Her last purchase was a pair of black stockings and a suspender belt.

Finally she prepared a three-course-meal that was a tribute to her ingenuity and determination. The first course was simple avocado and nutmeg. The second course was beefurgers with an avocado and nutmeg salad. The third course was avocado and nutmeg topped with whipped, artificial cream and glâcé cherries.

All in all, it was an ordered and planned assault that made Rommel's campaign in the desert look chaotic. As Malcolm brushed the last whisk of cream from his chin Joyce sat back to wait in a mood that can only be described as quietly and expectantly confident.

Unhappily, however, at just about the moment when Joyce was expecting to be putting up a little token resistance, she found herself standing outside the bathroom door while Malcolm, on the other side of the door, emitted the groans and whimpers of a man in torment. Shy as ever, he had been too embarrassed to tell her that he was allergic to avocado pears.

Joyce gave up the struggle shortly after that; she was somewhat consoled a little later when she heard that Malcolm had run off with a fifteen year old boy scout.

THE POWER HOUSE
Honey and marshmallow

Source and preparation

Honey is one of the most popular and effective aphrodisiac foods. It has been known for centuries that, if taken regularly, it will enhance desire and improve capacity. Taken by itself, however, honey is a fairly mild aphrodisiac. A much greater result can be obtained if it is mixed with a little ginger or pepper and then smeared liberally onto a marshmallow cube.

This mixture was first used about a hundred and fifty years ago by Jamaican women who somehow knew that the preparation could have a dramatic effect on their lives. Presumably, some local substitute for marshmallow was employed. According to traditional Jamaican legends, the mixture has always been used by women whose appetites are a little stronger than average. In the famous Philtre Papers, which were published about thirty years ago by a well known Swedish anthropologist, the source of this legend was traced back to 15th century Spain. It seems quite possible that the trick was carried over to Jamaica by one of the explorers who followed Columbus.

Type of effect

A honey and ginger soaked marshmallow will increase the rate at which blood flows into the veins and to help keep them enlarged for long periods of time.

Veins all over the body are affected, but it is the effect on the veins which supply the male organ and the tissues immediately around the vagina which give the honey and marshmallow mixture its rare qualities as an aphrodisiac. As far as both men and women are concerned the Power House has a dramatic value. The effect is basically to P.L.E.A.S.E. but the mixture will also produce a S.Q.U.E.A.L. in many cases.

Speed and length of action

The strengthening of the male organ and the softening of the complementary female parts, the two dominant qualities of the Power House aphrodisiac, begin within about half an hour and reach a peak within ninety minutes. The honey soaked marshmallow shouldn't be chewed for too long, since the enzymes present in saliva can have a damaging effect on the honey and marshmallow mixture.

Warning

Because the honey and marshmallow mixture produces a generalised peripheral vaso-dilatation, users often notice that they feel warm and look red. These modest and harmless side effects can occasionally be accompanied by more serious problems, for the general dilation of the veins means that there can be a central effect on the heart and blood pressure. It is therefore important that individuals with heart or circulation problems should not use the Power House without checking with their doctors first.

Some people who have used the Power House regularly for long periods of time have reported a higher than average incidence of varicose veins. Research is still going on to investigate the real relationship between the aphrodisiac and the disorder.

One final point worth making is that a honey and ginger soaked marshmallow will be rich in calories. Slimmers and others watching their weight should remember this and use the Power House sparingly.

Sweet dreams

I first heard about the unique values of a honey and ginger soaked marshmallow when I was working as a part time Assistant Medical Officer at a Family Planning Clinic in a small town in the North of England. The clinic was run by a privately financed charity and those of us working there were encouraged to provide a whole range of services from simple, straightforward contraceptive advice to marriage-guidance and sexual counselling.

I can still remember the day I first came across the Power House. It was a Wednesday in early summer and the sort of pleasant day that you wish could go on for ever. It hadn't been too hot even in the middle of the day and as the evening approached the temperature became just about perfect.

We'd seen about half a dozen clients when a woman in her late twenties came in to have a new Dutch cap fitted. They're a bit out of fashion today but then they were still quite popular. The West Indian nurse who worked with me in the clinic had helped the woman undress and was sorting through the drawer full of different caps when suddenly and quite unexpectedly the

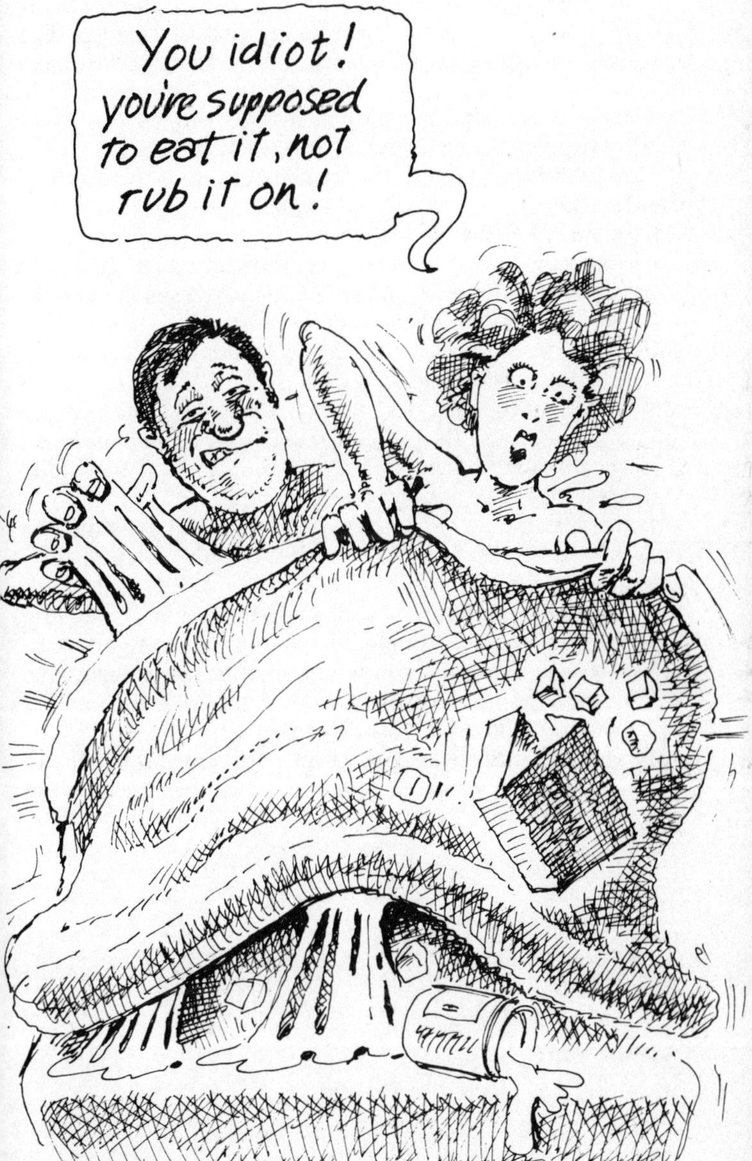
You idiot! you're supposed to eat it, not rub it on!

woman began to cry. 'I really don't know why I'm bothering with this,' she sobbed. Naturally, we invited her to tell us more.

With tears rolling down her cheeks and her whole body shaking with sadness the woman told us that her husband had been unfaithful to her so often that she'd lost count of the times.

'It's always young girls,' she explained. 'Always girls of sixteen and seventeen. And they've got to be virgins.'

'Why virgins?' asked the nurse, genuinely puzzled.

'He's not very well built,' the woman explained. 'If you know what I mean.'

We assured her that we knew what she meant.

The woman, having relieved herself of her secret, collapsed into another lengthy series of sobs. Finally, she shook her head and raised herself up slightly from the couch.

'Do you think if I had plastic surgery that things would be any better?' she wanted to know.

'You don't need to do anything that drastic,' smiled my Jamaican nurse. And she proceeded to tell our client to go home and prepare some honey-soaked marshmallows. I was quite astonished, but she was very serious about it.

'You give him two of those every evening and you take two yourself,' she insisted, 'and he'll think you've been shrink-wrapped onto him.'

The woman was almost pitifully grateful, but I was very sceptical. I didn't say anything, but to be honest I felt a bit cross. I thought the nurse had been wrong to offer the woman hope when there clearly wasn't any remote chance that such an old wives' tale could possibly work. I was wrong.

Six weeks later the woman was back in the clinic with a broad grin on her face. It was the first time I'd ever seen a Dutch cap completely worn out.

AFTERNOON TEA
Cannabis

Source and preparation

Next to alcohol, cannabis is the most widely used recreational drug in the world. It is sometimes thought of as a recent addition to the auto-therapeutic armoury but it has, in fact, been an extremely popular aphrodisiac for many centuries.

According to one old Arabian legend, a gentleman called Abdul Haylukh maintained an erection for thirty days after smoking hashish, while another Arab called Abdul Hayjeh is credited with having deflowered eighty virgins during one night after a few pipes of the substance.

Marco Polo tells the story of a sect called the Assassins, whose leader maintained power over his followers by giving them hashish to smoke and dancing girls to keep them company. Believing that the experiences they enjoyed during their drugged hours in the company of the expense account houris were merely a taste of heavenly things to come, the agents would risk anything asked of them.

Many of those who use hash or marijuana for its sexually stimulating properties may not be aware of the differences between the various types of preparation of this plant. It is important to understand that marijuana is the dried leaves of the plant, whereas hash (which is ten times as potent) is the resinous exudate that is scraped from the leaves.

Hash oil – five times as potent again as hash – contains an extraordinarily high content of tetrahydrocannabinol; it is prepared by boiling the powdered leaves of the plant in alcohol, straining the mixture, and then leaving it so that the alcohol will evaporate.

Another fact not commonly understood is that the best type of aphrodisiac effect is obtained from mature female marijuana plants which have not been pollinated. These are the source of the most exquisite effects.

It's obvious, then, that anyone seeking a useful sexual effect from cannabis should look for hash oil which has been obtained from a mature, unpollinated female plant. The oil should be burned in a small spoon and the vapour inhaled.

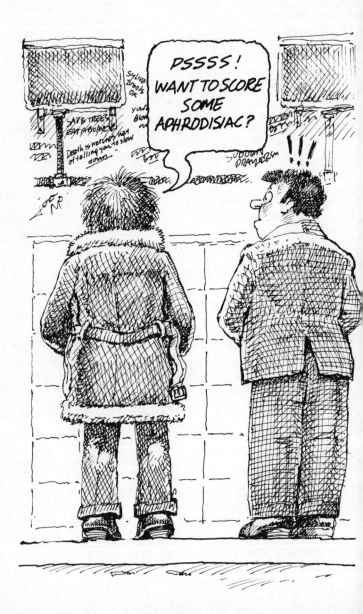

Type of effect

Marijuana and the other cannabis derivatives have a number of effects on those who use it. Its basic effect is to alter perception and to enhance and concentrate impulses and feelings. It does help break down some inhibitions but has remarkably little effect on those who are unwilling to experiment or risk new experiences. It's important to remember that cannabis is quite as likely to exaggerate feelings of distaste as those of love and affection.

This particular aphrodisiac is most suitable for individuals who already have willing partners but who are looking for new joys and greater peaks of performance. Although there is a modest S.I.N. factor the main effect is as a Moment of Response Extender.

Speed and length of action

Afternoon Tea derives its name from the fact that if evening action is required the drug ought to be used during the afternoon since an improvement in the quality of the sexual experience will usually take five or six hours to develop. Although slow to build the result is often prolonged. Love-making sessions can continue for two to three days after a particularly good bunch of grass has been used.

Warning

Men who use cannabis regularly sometimes notice that their breasts enlarge. This side effect is strangely, and some would say unfortunately, absent among women although there is some slight evidence that women who use cannabis sources notice a tingling in their breasts which can heighten their own pleasure.

The Trainee Vicars' Tea Party

When I was a medical student the best parties were invariably those held at the local theology college. I always rather suspected that the students there were anxious to cram as much fun as possible into the months remaining before graduation. Most were only too well aware that for the average practising clergyman, an afternoon spent running a 'guess the weight of the cake' stall at the church fete is about as close to excitement as life is likely to get.

Whether or not there was any justification for that suspicion, their parties were always pretty invigorating. The students were particularly adept at thinking up new parlour games and doing remarkably imaginative things with dog collars and candles. I remember one unusually athletic theologian who was expelled after organising a nude tennis match between members of his college and novice nuns from a local seminary. The principal of the theology college confessed afterwards that he had watched the match for two and a half hours before deciding that he'd have to step in.

For nearly two terms there were parties at one of the residential colleges every Saturday and Sunday; they used to begin early on Saturday afternoons and continue until mid-afternoon on Sundays. They couldn't go on longer because the college principal always returned from his weekend break at about that time. In addition to the theology students and half a dozen medical students, there were a number of nurses and clerical groupies around. Men of the cloth always seem to attract women. I think that perhaps it is because some women see them in the same light as homosexuals – in need of saving or converting.

The last of those golden weekends started particularly well. Some of the trainee vicars had managed to acquire a supply of marijuana from a botany student. It was a boiling hot summer weekend and the sweet smell of burning grass mingled with the acrid odour coming from the summer bonfire which always seemed to be smouldering at the bottom of the college gardens.

There were huge French windows leading out from the common room onto a top lawn which was studded with croquet hoops; and by nine o'clock that Saturday evening there must have been twenty or thirty couples scattered around inside the common room and between the hoops on the grass. Most were beginning to feel the effects of the hash they'd been smoking and were energetically celebrating their love for one another and for the world in general.

I'll always remember that particular weekend not so much for the rich odour of pot or the chorus of love-cries as for one particular remark which I overheard later that night. John Talbot, a theology graduate who'd come back to spend the weekend with friends, was being looked after by two youngs girls who wore nothing but a single crucifix between them. John was beginning to show signs of fatigue and it was the girl with the crucifix who uttered the phrase that stuck in my mind. 'More tea, vicar?' she suggested with a beguiling mixture of innocence, hope and goodwill. Vicarage tea parties and church fêtes have never seemed quite the same since then.

OYSTER PARADE
Dopamine

Source and preparation

Much of what we know about sexual response chemistry concerns two chemicals called dopamine and serotonin. These are vital neuro-transmitters which help to govern brain activity and control sexual desires. Serotonin normally inhibits sexual activity while dopamine is known to increase it.

Research has shown that there are a large number of readily available foods which contain dopamine. Of these sources broad beans and oysters are the two most substantial. The dopamine in these foodstuffs is concentrated, chemically clean and unadulterated by the trace minerals which sometimes contaminate other edibles rich in dopamine.

The main disadvantage with these sources of dopamine is that they are almost always (unsurprisingly) eaten. This method of consumption is of little value because to be effective dopamine has to be introduced directly into the venous system (a hazardous procedure known as mainlining) or absorbed into the bloodstream through the mucous membranes. I recommend the second of these alternatives. The mucous membrane method is safe, effective, painless and only marginally slower than a direct intravenous infusion. The human body contains mucous membranes at three convenient sites: the mouth is one; the other two are well below mouth-level.

To increase blood dopamine levels a food dopamine source must be kept in close contact with the mucous membranes for between fifteen and twenty minutes. Although broad beans are high in dopamine, most people find vegetables aesthetically unsuitable for the mucous membrane method and prefer to use oysters. The oysters need no special preparation and should simply be placed in contact with an appropriate membrane in groups of three or four. Some couples consider site selection an essential prelude to good lovemaking.

Type of effect

Dopamine has a very broad spectrum of activity and can improve desire, performance and the quality of the orgasm. It has no S.I.N. effect but does have G.O., S.T.A.R.T.,

P.L.E.A.S.E., M.O.R.E. and S.Q.U.E.A.L., properties. The value of the effect is much the same on men and women. Remember that although oysters do have a reputation as an aphrodisiac, it won't work unless they are allowed to remain in contact with a mucous membrane for the length of time noted above. Oysters swallowed quickly will be quite ineffectual.

Speed and length of action
Once the dopamine has been absorbed into the blood stream it has an almost immediate action on the brain. Sexual desire will reach a peak, and performance will be improved, in thirty minutes at most. The effect of the dopamine lasts for about eight hours and then slowly fades.

If this particular aphrodisiac is used regularly experiments will prove even more dramatic as time wears on. Dopamine has a cumulative strength and even though blood levels fall to a clinically insignificant level after about eight hours, enough dopamine remains in the blood stream to ensure that future oyster usage will have a much more interesting result.

Warning
The main danger with Oyster Parade lies in the fact that repeated application can lead to a dramatic increase in sexual activity. Individuals with weak hearts, poor general physiques or grumbling appendices should be wary of using this aphrodisiac more than once every six months. Individuals who are fit should be sure to allow a good deal of leisure time.

The Hallam Street secret
If a doctor runs away with a patient, seduces one in his consulting room or proves too enthusiastic when it comes to getting female patients to undress, then any complaint that is made will eventually find its way to a disciplinary body called the General Medical Council. This body has the responsibility of ensuring that doctors found guilty of unprofessional conduct will have their names removed from the register of approved practitioners. The popular press owes a great debt to the General Medical Council, since its hearings are usually open to reporters and the tabloids love risqué stories about doctors almost as much as the questionable carryings-on of scout masters or vicar's wives.

One case recently tried by the General Medical Council's disciplinary body was, however, so outrageous that it never

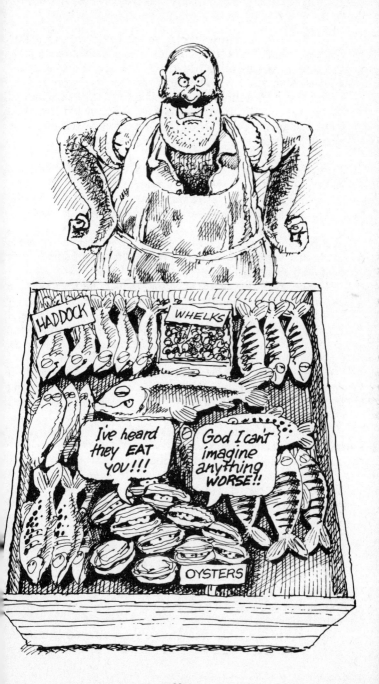

reached the popular newspapers. What happened apparently was that the editors of the country's leading daily journals were called to a meeting at the Council's headquarters where they were asked to make no reference in print to this particular case. To make sure the request was complied with, they were warned that if the story did appear, then the Council would approve a motion suggesting that all disciplinary cases in the future be held in camera.

The General Medical's Council's request didn't stem from any compassion for the doctor involved or even for his patients. Rather, it came as a result of the Council's belief that if the story became widely known there would be such an outcry that the status of the medical profession would be severely affected.

Having had access to these files, however, I feel that the details should be made public, principally because they provide a salutory warning about just how dangerous aphrodisiacs can be if used unwisely.

The person at the centre of this particular controversy was a gynaecologist who, for legal reasons, we had better refer to as Dr X. Although he had an honorary position at a leading general hospital Dr X's main income was provided by a consulting practice and it was his work in a private clinic which eventually attracted the attention of the General Medical Council.

For nearly a decade Dr X had specialised in the treatment of women who were suffering from sexual problems. Frigidity and loss of libido were the two symptoms which were mentioned most commonly in his consulting rooms but since women who have negligible libidos are unlikely to run much risk of becoming pregnant, he also saw a good number of patients who mistakenly thought themselves infertile.

When he first started in practice, Dr X used a variety of hormone treatments. Gradually, though, he grew more and more disillusioned with this type of therapy, believing its effectiveness to be limited.

Searching around for some more reliable way to help his patients, Dr X came across some early research work done by Professor Johnstone which showed the importance of dopamine levels in the blood. At about the same time, he happened to read the report which had demonstrated that oysters are dopamine-rich agents and therefore aphrodisiacal when placed in contact with the mucous membranes.

It was then that Dr X started to use oysters in a way which the General Medical Council later considered to be quite unprofessional. His technique was delightfully simple. When a patient complained of frigidity, anorgasmia or loss of libido he would perform what seemed a routine gynaecological examination, but would leave behind a pair of powerful Mediterranean oysters. Then he would give his patient an injection of distilled water and tell hcr to return in a week.

On the second visit most patients would happily confirm that they had enjoyed extremely successful sexual encounters within a short time of having the injection. They would also report that their libidos had since disappeared again. This meant that Dr X would have to perform another examination, replace the oysters with a fresh pair, and give the unsuspecting woman another injection of water.

Business went very well for Dr X and his practice blossomed. Six months after starting his special treatment he was looking after so many happy patients that a small fishing village in Southern Italy was supplying him with its entire weekly oyster catch.

In the end things went wrong simply because Dr X underestimated the power of his treatment. It was not until later that researchers discovered that blood dopamine levels can be raised to extraordinarily high levels by the repeated use of oysters. Instead of suffering from anorgasmia and frigidity, many of Dr X's patients became over-demanding and sexually aggressive. And that, in turn, meant that their husbands, boyfriends and lovers often found themselves physically unable to meet their demands. Tragically, thirty-four of Dr X's first hundred and fifty patients were widows within six months of starting the treatment; another nineteen had suffered the loss of lovers, boyfriends and formerly reliable tradesmen.

The occurrence of these apparently inexplicable events among patients from a single practice – allied with a great deal of professional jealousy surrounding Dr X's success – meant that a report to the General Medical Council was inevitable. Prevented from practising by the disciplinary body, Dr X retired to the same Italian village which he had kept in employment for so many months. Rumour has it that the village people are rich, happy and multiplying fast.

BONE SHAKER
Satyrion

Source and preparation

Anyone preparing a scientific study of available aphrodisiacs has to struggle to differentiate between the real and the imagined, the factual and the mythical, the genuine and the spurious. The literature relating to this branch of sexual chemistry contains such a confusing mixture of solid, objective advice and flimsy, subjective fantasy that the value of some substances said to be aphrodisiacal is difficult to determine.

Of all reported aphrodisiacs the one which has spawned more stories than any other is satyrion: a mysterious and apparently powerful substance which was mentioned more frequently even than the seemingly ubiquitous mandrake in the erotic writings of Greek and Roman authors. Hercules is said to have deflowered all fifty daughters of his host Thespius when given a single dose of this powerful drug. Proculus is reputed to have initiated over 100 virgins in 15 days. And another, anonymous, hero is said to have successfully enjoyed 70 *successive* instances of coitus. Described by one author as being so powerful that it could arouse sexual passion simply by being held in the hand, satyrion led to the production and dissemination of a veritable library of stories and anecdotes. Even Pliny wrote about it, suggesting that one might eat lettuce in order to cool off and reduce the excessive lust sometimes produced by the drug.

Like many others, I was sceptical about these claims, particularly since I was unable to identify satyrion as a known or available plant. Indeed, I was about to banish the substance to the drawer in which I have filed those supposed aphrodisiacs about which there is more legend than fact, when I discovered that an English botanist called Shaw had finally identified satyrion as being orchis mascula, a wild woodland orchid, better known as the 'early purple orchid'.

Professor Howard B. Johnstone, of the Institute of Sexual Chemistry in Maryland, has already performed preliminary experimental work with orchis mascula and his studies suggest that satyrion's extraordinary reputation was by no means an exaggeration. Using an ancient Greek recipe which suggested that satyrion worked best when tossed off in a libation of goat' milk, Johnstone and his co-workers have shown that the tuber of the orchis mascula needs only to be dipped into a glass of milk in order to turn the beverage into an immensely powerful aphrodisiac.

Type of effect
Satyrion (or orchis mascula as we now know it to be) has a very general aphrodisiac action although, surprisingly perhaps, it seems to have virtually no effect as a disinhibitor. It has an arousing effect, an impressive effect on performance and a valuable influence on orgasmic quality. It has G.O., S.T.A.R.T., P.L.E.A.SE., M.O.R.E., and S.Q.U.E.A.L. properties.

Speed and length of action
Satyrion begins to work almost instantaneously and reaches a peak within one or two minutes. The length of the effect depends directly upon the amount of satyrion absorbed into the body. When a tuber has simply been dipped into a glass of milk the effect can be over within a matter of minutes. However, if a more substantial quantity is consumed the effect can last for hours or even – according to reliable reports – for days.

Warning
The speed with which satyrion works should never be under-estimated. Professor Johnstone recommends that those intending to use it should undress before they take the aphrodisiac in order to avoid damage to clothing. His research assistants have discovered that they have to wear heavy-duty rubber gloves when handling the roots. Botanists collecting the plant have reported some appallingly embarrassing experiences.

Natural justice
Edwina Shaw enjoyed the company of plants in the same way that other women enjoy the company of friends and neighbours. She talked to them and confided in them, she argued with them and she shared with them her loves, her fears and her aspirations. It had been the same for as long as she could remember. At school when the other girls were drooling over photographs of James Dean, Elvis Presley and Bill Haley, she would be gazing with equally sincere admiration at engravings of rare botanical specimens. While the others were bopping and jiving at the

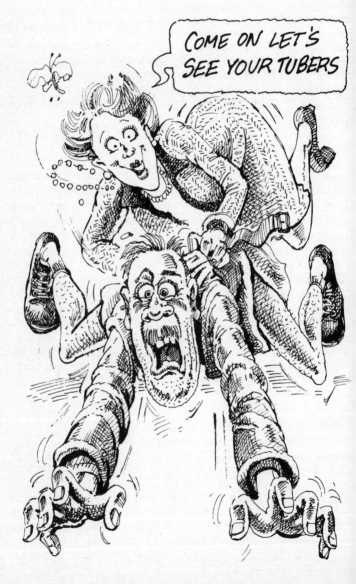

church hall she would be peering down a microscope. And while her classmates were secretly meeting their boyfriends behind the bicycle sheds, she'd be searching for rare ivy behind the sports pavilion. Friends might save up to buy lipsticks, eye-shadow and ear rings; Edwina would save for dissecting instruments, magnifying glasses and collecting equipment. She wasn't an ugly girl – in fact she was more than ordinarily pretty – but given the choice of a pair of nylons and a new botany textbook, she'd have chosen the textbook every time.

No one had been very surprised when she'd been awarded a university scholarship nor had anyone at the university been taken aback when she'd won just about every major prize. Plants were both her vocation and her hobby.

After she obtained her doctorate Miss Shaw was made Assistant Lecturer in the University Botany department. It wasn't an appointment that involved a great deal of lecturing and so she was encouraged by her professor to select a subject for more postgraduate work. After searching through the academic journals for a couple of months she eventually decided to try and identify some of the plants discussed in Greek and Roman literature. One of the plants she decided to try and identify was satyrion: mentioned frequently in classical literature as a powerful aphrodisiac. Thus far, modern botanists had been unable to isolate it.

So it was that when this thirty-three year old botanist, bespectacled and draped in the shapeless tweeds and useful brogues which are the traditional rural uniform of the female academic, happened to chance upon a variety of orchis mascula in a remote corner of a Suffolk woodland, and saw that it matched the description of satyrion quite perfectly, she was filled with a keen sense of professional delight. Crick and Watson, having unravelled the mysteries of the DNA molecule, could hardly have been more excited.

The plant lay half-buried between the roots of a dying elm. At first Miss Shaw did nothing but gaze with admiration at the perfectly formed petals of the purple flowers. Then, knowing that in order to identify the plant as satyrion she would have to take it back to the university, photograph it, draw it, and record its every measurement, she carefully clawed the earth away from the plant's subterranean tubers. Within minutes she'd scooped away enough earth to free the plant. She held her find carefully and studied it for a moment or two.

The simple and relatively uncomplicated act of lifting the

plant from the ground was, for Miss Shaw, the beginning of a new life. Within seconds of touching the pale tubers, she began to feel a surge of passion in her loins the like of which she had never known before. By the time she realised exactly what was happening, and had thrust the satyrion deep inside her specimen bag, it was too late. Consumed by a powerful, natural lust she set off back along the path through the woods.

On many days she could have walked for miles without encountering a soul, but as luck would have it she met someone walking towards her when she was still half-a-mile from the road. It was a man, dressed in a long, shabby raincoat, and as she approached he suddenly pulled the two unbuttoned sides of the garment apart to reveal what looked, to Miss Shaw, remarkably like the tuber of her satyrion plant.

The flasher had adopted the woods as his regular patch some months before and had spent a good deal of time plodding through the bracken and exposing himself to nature-lovers, ornithologists, ramblers, girl-guides and the like. He knew what reaction to expect – or *thought* he knew. When the wretched man saw the tweed-clad figure of Miss Shaw running towards him at top speed he simply did not know what to do. Like a rabbit caught in the glare of a car's headlights he stood unmoving and terrified.

It was at first an unpromising and clumsy coupling but after Miss Shaw had thrust the satyrion's tubers into the terrified hands of the unfortunate flasher things went from strength to strength. With the two of them fired by the power of the world's most potent aphrodisiac, the woodlands reverberated to their cries and groans. The satyrion had changed Miss Shaw's life for ever. Of the flasher, there are no reliable reports.

NUTS IN MAY
Horse chestnuts

Source and preparation

The Marquis de Sade was the first writer in modern times to comment on the fact that the blossom of the horse chestnut tree smells very much like human semen but this fact had, of course, been common knowledge for centuries. Some observers have suggested that Socrates, who was particularly fond of outdoor tutorials, would try to make sure that he sat underneath a chestnut tree while lecturing to his students. A small forest of these trees still stands on the Island of Cos where Hippocrates is said to have practised during his early years as a physician.

The reason for the similarity puzzled scientists for many centuries until it was discovered that both semen and the horse chestnut blossom contain a unique combination of a fibrinogen like protein and an acid-soluble phosphorus consisting mainly of phosphorylcholine and glyerylphosophorylcholine. When these substances were mixed artificially in a laboratory at the Institute for Botanical Research in Wellington, New Zealand scientists found that the olfactory sensation was indistinguishable from that obtained from semen or horse chestnut blossom.

Preparing an aphrodisiac from horse chestnut blossom is very easy, particularly since the blossoms can be safely and effectively stored in a deep freeze for up to twelve months.

It is possible to manufacture perfumes from the blossom by compressing the flowers and using a fatty oil to extract the fibrinogen and acid-soluble phosphorus. Most of those who favour Nuts in May have, however, discovered that it is not even necessary to do this.

The simplest method is to put a small handful of blossom into a muslin bag and to tie the bag onto the hot water tap when taking a bath, placing it in such a way that the hot water has to run through the muslin. In this way the bath water can be infused with the scent of the flowers and in due course the bather will leave the room in a heady cloud of natural perfume.

Type of effect

Nuts in May has an effect only on women, window dressers and some male hairdressers. It has powerful G.O. and S.T.A.R.T.

effects and a useful if modest S.I.N. effect too.

Speed and length of action
The odour of the horse chestnut blossom tends to linger for hours, and once a susceptible individual comes within range the impact is usually instantaneous.

Warning
It is important to remember that the potency of Nuts in May can be felt accidentally if a woman lingers near a horse chestnut tree in blossom. Women on picnics, for example, have often found themselves aroused unexpectedly, while others, shopping in towns with tree lined avenues perhaps, might well be seen to blush for no apparent reason.

The spreading chestnut trees

One of the first medical jobs I ever had was as an assistant to a G.P. who had a practice in one of those small market towns in central England which are not quite sure whether to allow themselves to be dragged out of the nineteenth century.

There were, it is true, some signs of progress though not very welcome ones. A large car-component factory had been built at one side of the town and a small industrial estate shared its access roads with a new housing complex. There was a large multi-storey hotel too, built by an American chain that seemed to have beds available all over the world. The town was populated by a mixture of car workers and their families and elderly, retired colonels and their ladies.

The general practitioner for whom I was working was, in his own way, a good example of the dichotomy that existed in the town. A few bits and pieces of modern medical equipment demonstrated that he had at least one foot in the twentieth century, but he still set great store by the more old-fashioned methods.

He was, for instance, one of the last general practitioners to look after all his maternity patients without help from clinics. He was a great believer in encouraging women to have babies in the comfort of their own homes and genuinely enjoyed bringing babies into the world.

It was the obstetrics side of the practice that I still remember most vividly. When I joined him in January just a little more than ten years ago, I discovered to my amazement that no fewer

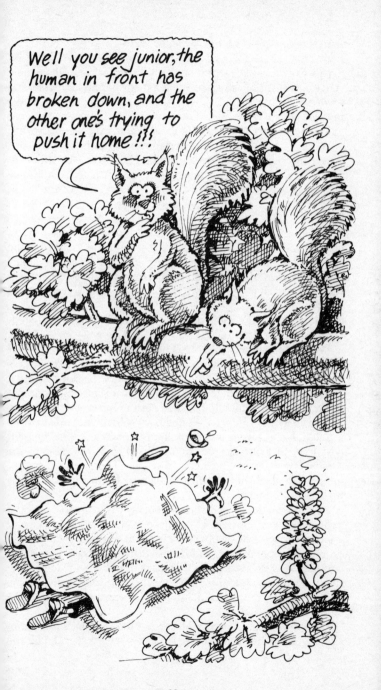

than twenty-nine of his patients were expecting babies in February. Since the average sort of medical practice would hardly expect to have that many new births in a year, that single statistic was quite astonishing. What was almost unbelievable was that twenty two of those twenty nine women lived in the same fairly short avenue. There were sixty houses in the road and just about every woman of child bearing age was pregnant.

When I remarked on this extraordinary statistic to my employer he seemed quite unsurprised. 'They have a lot of February babies in Dorset Avenue,' he confirmed. 'It's the horse chestnut trees.' I must have looked puzzled. 'There are lots of horse chestnut trees in Dorset Avenue,' he explained. 'They all blossom in May.'

When my expression clearly told him that I still didn't understand he went on to explain that he had noticed over the years that all the fertile women living in Dorset Avenue regularly conceived in May and delivered their babies in February.

'But what's it got to do with the horse chestnut trees?' I asked him.

The good doctor winked. 'You wait until May,' he insisted. 'You'll soon find out then.'

Well, the women in Dorset Avenue duly delivered their babies in February and with the hustle and bustle of late winter epidemics I completely forgot about the horse chestnut trees.

I forgot about them, that is, until they came into blossom that spring and I happened to park my car in Dorset Avenue on my way to visit one of February's newborn babies who had acquired a cough and a cold. It was then that I understood. The moment that I set foot outside my car I realised that the whole of the avenue smelt like a lovers' bedroom. There was a heavy, oppressive smell of sexuality in the air, so strong that it was impossible to ignore.

As I walked the short distance from my car to the front door of the house I was visiting, I could see that every door and every window in the street had been flung open. The young mothers of Dorset Avenue, dressed in their brightly coloured, low necked summer dresses, sat on their doorsteps or leaned out of bedroom windows, chatting and soaking up the sun; they smiled at me and waved as they waited impatiently for their husbands to come home.

It seemed clear that whether or not the husbands arrived in time, another batch of February babies would soon be on the way.

40

THE CLAYMORE
Parachlorophenylalanine

Source and preparation

The value of parachlorophenylalanine as an aphrodisiac was first discovered by accident when researchers in Italy who were using the drug as a headache remedy found that the sexual function of seventeen out of twenty-three patients improved dramatically.

Further studies done at a mid-western Pharmacology Department showed that parachlorophenylalanine is a potent inhibitor of tryptophan hydroxylase, itself a key enzyme involved in the production of serotonin. Serotonin is a drug produced within the human body; and it has a markedly repressive effect on sexuality. By interfering with the essential enzyme tryptophan the parachlorophenylalanine reduces the serotonin levels and thereby enhances the possibility of sexual activity.

The substance used in Italy was, of course, a synthetic compound prepared in a commercial laboratory and drug restrictions mean that, in most countries, it is unavailable without a doctor's prescription. However, it has been shown that parachlorophenylalanine occurs naturally in a number of unlikely sites. The most potent source is known to be the rearmost hump of the Bactrian camel, an animal found only in the highlands of central Asia.

Although evidence suggests that the levels of parachlorophenylalanine in the fat stores which make up the hump are fairly high at all times, it seems that the concentration of this useful aphrodisiac increases quite dramatically during the rutting season. Zoologists at a Scottish University, who have done some of the most important work on this subject, claim that the increase in the levels of circulating parachlorophenylalanine is responsible for the fits of rage which characterise the Bactrian camel in rut.

Concentrated and purified parachlorophenylalanine is relatively powerful and the normal dose of the synthetic drug is 15 mg per kilogram of body weight when taken orally. The concentrations in camel hump fat during rut are lower and 100 mg of fat is usually needed to provide a reasonable effect. Bactrian hump fat is obtainable from most high-class food stores.

Type of effect
Because it works directly on the serotonin levels, parachlor-ophenylalanine has an effect on sexual arousal and interest rather than performance. It works on both men and women and has G.O. and S.T.A.R.T. properties.

Speed and length of action
Parachlorophenylalanine usually takes seven to ten days to produce any result. Its presence becomes noticeable when the blood levels of circulating serotonin fall below a critical level. Those using this aphrodisiac have reported that the onset of the drug can be very dramatic and unexpected.

The potency of parachlorophenylalanine remains for six to seven hours but then fades quickly. The drug can, however, recur and some of those who use it regularly claim that after first taking parachlorophenylalanine, consequent sexual arousal can occur intermittently for some months afterwards.

Warning
It is important to be aware of the time delay between taking this aphrodisiac and experiencing any arousal. Users who have ignored this delay have been disappointed, frustrated and offended. On occasion even those who have been fully aware of the inevitable delay have found themselves suffering mentally as a direct consequence.

A good time coming
Melbourne, Australia 7.30 am Thursday

Bernard Williamson handed his passport and his ticket to the counter clerk at the Qantas desk with a feeling of considerable relief. He'd been travelling across Australia for nearly a month and although he had successfully negotiated the sale of several million pounds' worth of computer equipment, he was glad the trip was nearly over. He was tired and he wanted to go home: back to Surrey where a spacious, five bedroomed house, a swimming pool and a gorgeous blonde wife were waiting for him. He had one more call to make, at the Hong Kong office of an international data processing agency, and then he could look forward to spending a week at home – most of it, he mused, in bed. He and Wilma had a lot of time to make up.

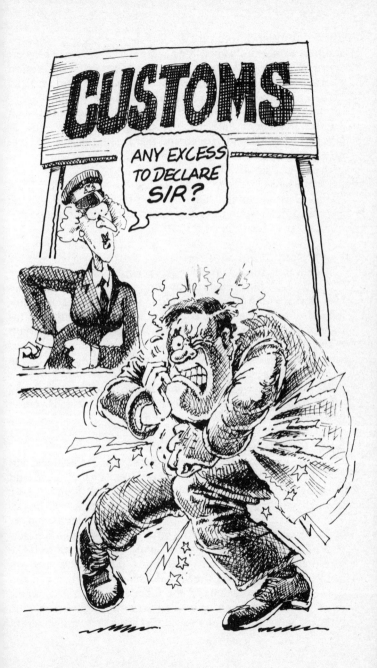

43

Surrey, England 9.30 pm Wednesday

While her husband waited for his flight at Melbourne airport, Wilma Williamson was struggling to concentrate on a television play. It wasn't a particularly bad play but the hero and the heroine had already made love three times and Wilma didn't think she could cope if they did it again. She looked at the clock for the umpteenth time that day. Bernard was due home at 5.30 pm on Sunday afternoon and that meant that she had just ninety-two hours to wait. Four more nights in an empty bed with cool silk sheets.

On the screen the hero was taking his shirt off again. The hairs on his chest reminded her of Bernard. She reached for the remote control switch resting on the arm of her chair and turned him into an advertisement for cat food.

Hong Kong, 1 am Saturday

The man from the data processing agency seemed fascinated by the stripper's skills. He'd never seen ping pong balls travel so fast. Bernard found it all very routine. In the course of entertaining out-of-town clients, he had spent half his life in night clubs watching girls take off their clothes and do strange things with unusual props. These days he often found himself more fascinated by the reactions of those who were with him than by the activities of the entertainers.

He wondered what Wilma was doing. He hoped she'd remembered to lay in plenty of champagne and caviar. He could feel the first stirrings of desire in his loins.

Surrey, England 5 pm Friday

It had been just five days ago when Bernard had telephoned and told her that he'd be home on Sunday. His plane was due to land at three and it usually took him two-and-a-half hours to pass through customs, collect his baggage and get a taxi home. They'd taken their parachlorophenylalanine tablets together, both chewing toffees to hide the bitter taste of the aphrodisiac.

With forty-eight hours to go Wilma was checking to make sure that she'd remembered everything. The black nightgown he liked was draped over the bedside chair, there was caviar and champagne in the 'fridge and the Allansons, who usually came round to use the swimming pool on Sundays, had been asked to come on Saturday instead. Now it was just a matter of waiting.

Heathrow, London 3 pm Sunday

The 'plane had landed exactly on time. Bernard felt very pleased with himself. He'd travelled half way round the world, done another half a million pounds' worth of business in Hong Kong, and had managed to keep to his schedule without a moment's delay. He could already feel the powerful effects of the para-chlorophenylalanine fortifying a natural desire to be back with his wife. He and Wilma had used the aphrodisiac regularly for two years. They found that it gave their lovemaking an edge and a force which carried them both to heights of ardour, passion and physical excitement which most people assume cannot exist outside the novels of D.H. Lawrence. With two hours to go, Bernard was aware of the mild burning sensation which told him that the drug was working.

Limping slightly he made his way across the tarmac and into the carousel area to collect his baggage. Together with the other passengers from his flight, he waited impatiently for his suit-cases to arrive.

Surrey, England 3.45 pm Sunday

The parachlorophenylalanine was working well. Wilma was beginning to ache with desire. She'd changed into her night-gown at 3.30 just in case the 'plane was a few minutes early. And now she was sitting in the living room waiting for the next hour-and-three-quarters to disappear. She felt hot and a little feverish.

Heathrow, London 4.00 pm Sunday

The baggage still had not been unloaded from the aeroplane. Twice Bernard had asked the official who stood at the entrance to the customs point if he could go through and leave his luggage behind. Twice they'd told him that it wasn't allowed. They said that since he had admitted to having luggage he would have to wait and collect it before he could leave the area.

Surrey, England 4.45 pm Sunday

Wilma had flung her nightgown aside and was stretched out, naked, on the bed. She'd taken the telephone off the hook and put two bottles of champagne into an ice bucket. She was ripe for loving.

Heathrow, London 5.00 pm Sunday

There was a rumour that the baggage handlers had walked out

and were refusing to offload any more luggage. The carousel was still and silent. Bernard was standing in a corner where he could keep an eye on the conveyor belt; he was trying as best he could to hide the plain evidence of near-ungovernable lust; he felt as if he might explode at any minute. Although the other passengers, once restive and belligerent, had now adopted the stuporous attitude of frustrated travellers everywhere, Bernard was growing more tense by the second. He found himself studying the other passengers with ravenous sexual hunger.

Surrey, England 7.00 pm Sunday

The parachlorophenylalanine had done its job to perfection. For two hours Wilma, loaded to the point of pain with an immense charge of sexual energy, had been fighting her frustration. When the doorbell rang, it didn't occur to her to wonder why her husband should ring the bell to his own house; she raced downstairs and had the door open before the sound of the chimes had died away.

The policeman who had called to inform her that Bernard had been arrested at the airport for rape, was trouserless and flat on his back on the garden path before he'd even had time to remove his helmet. It was a unique case: a double rape by members of the same household; and particularly notable for the fact that one was a woman. The Sunday press had a field-day, of course. They seemed particularly intrigued by the fact that both defendants cited the use of an aphrodisiac as part of their defence. The judge, unsurprisingly, was not impressed.

EASTERN PROMISE
Ginseng

Source and preparation

Ginseng has a long tradition as an aphrodisiac in China. Although most westerners believe that the various forms of ginseng have very similar properties, the Chinese favour different varieties in much the same sort of way that connoisseurs favour particular wines. Those practised in the selection and use of ginseng claim that the most powerful aphrodisiac action is obtained from the variety that grows wild in Manchuria. Much of the ginseng sold commercially today is grown in the Eastern United States, Canada, Korea, India and Southern China; but experts at the Peking School of Pharmacology consider those roots to be significantly inferior to roots from the Manchurian plain.

This remarkably fertile area is surrounded on three sides by mountains but on the south is open to the gentle breezes from the Yellow Sea and the Gulf of Chihli. It seems that this unique combination of geographical and meteorological circumstances explains the unequalled value of the ginseng from this area.

The most expensive Manchurian roots are, naturally, those which most closely resemble the human form. Tubers which have testis-like protruberances are widely sought by those who seek to benefit from the root's value as an aphrodisiac.

It really does not matter precisely how the root is prepared for consumption. Some Chinese users believe that it should be smoked, others like to make it into a thick tea; then there's a school of thought that claims that the strongest possible result is obtained if the root is chewed.

Type of effect

The consequence of ingesting ginseng is almost entirely physical. It improves the stamina, strength and power of those who take it and so has general P.L.E.A.S.E. qualities. Ginseng is not suitable for those who wish to improve their partner's compliance, nor is it of any value to those who suffer from repressions and inhibitions. It is only of use to those whose physical capabilities do not match their mental ambitions.

ONE THOUSAND MILLION CHINESE CAN'T BE WRONG!!!

(Correct on going to press!)

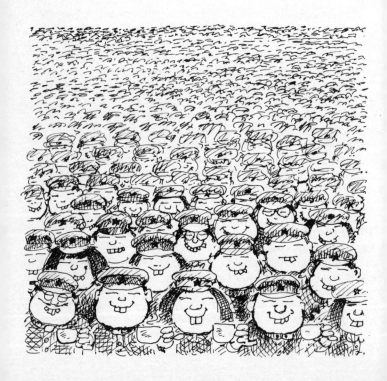

48

Speed and length of action

Ginseng is one of the slowest acting aphrodisiacs. It takes seven or eight hours for the drug to work. It is also one of the longest acting aphrodisiacs and users have claimed that the results are still apparent eight to ten days after the consumption of a single root.

Warning

A minor hazard with ginseng has been the reported incidence of breast development in males who take it frequently. This phenomenon is rarely found among female users, but a number of men who have been enthusiastic believers in the power of ginseng have abandoned the substance when their breast development reached embarrassing proportions.

Much more important than this, however, is that (according to research done in Russia) there is a considerable risk that those who use ginseng will push themselves beyond the limits of their physical endurance. One published report showed that eleven out of sixteen men who had regularly used ginseng as an aphrodisiac had died in bed but not alone!

Deidre's Good Buy

I'll never forget the first few months I spent in the village where I now practise. I arrived at about the same time as the new vicar who brought with him a pretty, likeable and enthusiastic young wife, who took her role in life very seriously. Deidre and Cuthbert had only been married a month and she still got quite a thrill when people called her Mrs Fording. Her husband only had a small village church to look after but Deidre couldn't have been prouder if he'd been an Archbishop with a cathedral of his own.

Naturally, she had a number of practical responsibilities as the wife of the community's only clergyman, and from the beginning she was determined to ensure that she managed her semi-ecumenical tasks with diligence, skill and a clear eye for detail. She didn't want anyone saying nasty things about her or blackening her husband's reputation because of something she had done – or had left undone.

One of her jobs was to provide the refreshments for all the meetings which were held in the church hall, the vestry and the vicarage. There was the weekly sewing meeting every Monday, the choir practice on Tuesdays and Thursdays, the church council on every third Tuesday, the Women's Institute on Wednesdays, the Young Wives' group on every second Thursday, the scouts on those Thursdays when the Young Wives weren't meeting, the girl guides on alternative Fridays and the bellringers on Fridays and Saturdays.

Deidre didn't have to prepare anything special for any of these meetings but it was customary for the vicar's wife to provide a pot of tea and a tin of biscuits. Now, providing a supply of tea and biscuits may not sound much of a responsibility but when you're living on the very limited stipend allotted to a rural clergyman and you've got to purchase enough tea and biscuits for dozens of visitors each week, the cost of the tea alone can take up a significant part of your weekly budget. It was, therefore, as an economy measure that Deidre decided to buy her supplies as cheaply as possible; and I suppose that simple and honest sense of economy, allied to her youth and inexperience, led her to purchase a twenty-six-pound catering pack of ginseng tea that the owner of the local village store happened to be anxious to unload at a bargain price.

To begin with, one or two of the villagers found the tea that was being served at the vicarage rather odd. Some members of the sewing circle were a little critical. But Deidre was a pleasant young woman and no-one wanted to hurt her feelings, so they said nothing. And since the aphrodisiac effect of ginseng develops very slowly and produces nothing more than an improvement in the physical capacities of those who enjoy it, none of Deidre's guests associated the tea with the improved quality of their sex lives.

In the weeks following my arrival as a young general practitioner in the village, I was astonished to find just how many sexually related disorders there were among the villagers. I had to deal with an extraordinary number of patients with backache, many cases of young ladies with 'honeymoon cystitis', a significant rise in unexpected pregnancies among the girl guides, and all sorts of other problems most regularly associated with rather too-enthusiastic love-making.

I was beginning to think that there must be some secret ingredient in the village air or water and wondered just how long it took to influence the behaviour of newcomers. The mystery was solved, however, when I had to call round to see young Deidre Fording who had just found out that she was pregnant.

After I'd finished examining her she insisted on making me a cup of tea; and while I was watching her prepare it I realised that if I'd been a more assiduous member of the church, then I might not have had to wait until the hereafter to experience heavenly bliss.

I didn't have the heart to tell Deidre what she'd been doing to the village. Fortunately, (or unfortunately) it was a short-lived event because a couple of weeks later the supply of cheap ginseng tea ran out; and the complaints my patients brought to the surgery were evidence that 'normal servicing' had been resumed.

BANANA SURPRISE
Bufotenine

Source and preparation

When Columbus sailed back to Europe in the late fifteenth century, one of the substances he carried with him was cohoba, a type of snuff that had for many years been particularly popular in Haiti – popular because of its well-proven properties as an aphrodisiac. Cohoba was not properly analysed until the 1950s when a German chemist working in Colorado discovered that its active ingredient was a substance called bufotenine. This was identified as an hallucinogenic alkaloid, known to occur in a number of other natural substances. It is, for example, present in small quantities in rabbits' lungs, the skins of toads and the mushroom *amanita muscaria*. (The present of bufotenine in toad skin might well explain why it was a popular ingredient in so many witches' brews and why so many fairy stories seem to involve toads and beautiful princesses.)

The richest natural source of bufotenine is not, however, any of these exotica, but the common banana skin which contains something like seven times as much of the drug per milligram as any other naturally-occurring substance. Stewed, sieved and turned into a thin soup – which can be served either hot or cold – banana skin is one of the most important and widely available of all aphrodisiacs.

When the high bufotenine content of banana skin was first identified back in the 1950s, its use became so widespread that the Federal Drug Authority was apparently instructed by an aide of the then President of the United States to produce a report condemning it as potentially dangerous. The President's advisers were afraid that if the unusual qualities associated with banana skin became too widely known, the population control plan (then in its infancy) would be, as it were, stillborn.

The report proved extremely effective and today banana skins are used only by a very small number of knowing individuals.

Type of effect

Bufotenine acts in a simple and straightforward way on sexual activity. It has G.O., S.T.A.R.T., M.O.R.E., and S.Q.E.A.L. properties and is most suitable for individuals whose capabilities do not match up to their intentions.

Speed and length of action
Bufotenine begins to work about four hours after it is first taken into the digestive system. For late evening activity it should be consumed at about 7 pm. The effect lasts for between 6 and 8 hours.

Warning
Anyone using bufotenine must be fit. As a general rule those who cannot run a six-minute mile should avoid Banana Surprise.

The secret success of the Lover's Nest

Back in the late 1950s, Arnold and Thelma Lodge had a small restaurant in New York called *The Lover's Nest*. The restaurant had no more than a dozen tables and it was situated in one of the least fashionable parts of the west side. It certainly didn't look the sort of place likely to pose a major threat to the city's trendier eating establishments.

Oddly, it was the restaurant's lack of reputation and un-classy location which helped to make it a modest success. Because it was away from the main-stream of New York social life, it became a meeting-place for those citizens conducting secret affairs and arranging clandestine meetings. Politicians took their mistresses there and journalists used the place to meet their 'secret sources'. No one at *The Lover's Nest* ever spoke in anything louder than a whisper.

Conscious of the needs of their clientele, Arnold and Thelma Lodge had, over the years, arranged the restaurant's decor with a special regard for confidentiality. The lighting was dim; all the tables were enclosed by tiny, private cubicles; the waiters were discreet; and the restaurant had two quite different entrances so that couples could arrive and leave separately.

For six or seven years the restaurant remained modestly successful and enabled its owners to enjoy a comfortable if not extravagant lifestyle. There were very few evenings when they were not fully booked and to get a table on a weekday (when the demand for that very exclusive type of restaurant facility is at its highest) diners had to book several weeks in advance.

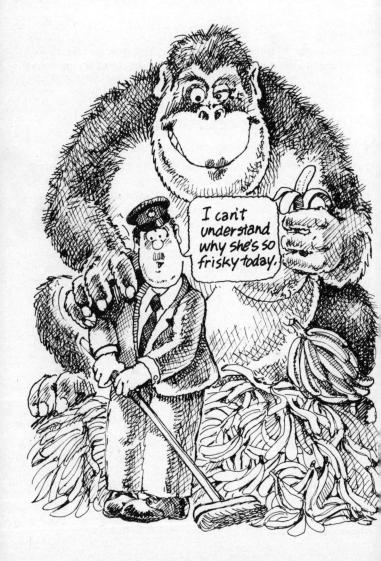

The character and success of the restaurant remained un-changed until the Lodges hired a new chef. The man they appointed to the post was young, ambitious and enthusiastic. Before he consented to work at *The Lover's Nest* he persuaded the owners to pay him a share of the profits rather than a fixed salary. The Lodges thought this an unusual arrangement but one that seemed to be to their advantage.

Within a few weeks of the new chef's appointment, *The Lover's Nest* became one of the most extraordinarily popular dining places in the city. The demand for tables grew at such an astonishing rate that the Lodges found themselves having to choose between opening an annexe and putting up their prices to discourage all but the wealthy. Since they had no wish to try and run a larger establishment they chose the easier solution and increased their charges threefold.

Of the relatively small number of dishes that the new chef created, by far the most successful was a special type of soup known simply as Potage de la Maison. This delicacy proved so popular as a first course choice that the Lodges gradually stopped offering alternative hors d'oeuvres. If you wanted to start a meal with pâté, whitebait, shrimps or melon you'd have to wait while the chef sent out to a nearby delicatessen.

The soup was so much in demand because it seemed to have a powerful and dramatic effect on the love-making ability of those who drank it. A meal at *The Lover's Nest* had always been considered an excellent start to a romantic evening; but a meal that started with a bowl of the restaurant's new soup was a prelude to a sexual symphony. Men whose normal capabilities were limited both in quality and quantity found themselves turning in performances they'd only ever dreamt of in their baths. Men in their sixties, seventies and eighties suddenly discovered that it was no longer just their wealth that attracted beautiful young women. An oil-billionaire in his seventies actually found himself fighting for the restaurant bill with a twenty year old model from a Manhattan advertising agency.

In the end, though, the restaurant's astonishing success led to its downfall. Finding themselves compared unfavourably with an eating house which most of them considered second-rate, four of New York's most fashionable restaurants hired a private detective agency to investigate *The Lover's Nest* and discover just what was proving such an attraction. The detective agency uncovered the fact that the chef was using banana skins in the preparation of his soup. And it was that same detective agency which, acting on the instructions of one of the city's most powerful restaurant chains, sent a copy of its report to the Federal Drug Authority and the city health department.

It would have been difficult, perhaps, to prove that anything criminal or dangerous to public health was involved. There are other ways of bringing pressure to bear – and paying to ensure that it *is* brought to bear – than through 'the proper channels'. Suffice it to say that a certain Italian brotherhood is not wholly unconnected with the New York catering business. At any rate, the Lodges closed their restaurant and left the city. Their clientele, needless to say, were devastated – though rumour has it that on the day of closing the chef offered to auction a popular recipe. Someone, somewhere, paid a quarter of a million dollars for it, or so the legend goes, and is embarked on a manufacturing programme that might well make prohibition seem a penny-ante game.

RAW PASSION
Steak tartare

Source and preparation

Steak tartare is widely recognised as a useful and effective aphrodisiac. Well-spiced, well-pounded and served with blood seeping out of the flesh, this dish is popular among experienced lovers all over the world. It provides fresh vigour, renewed sexual energy and exceptional staying power. As the indefatigable Dr Johnson once said to Boswell, 'there is nothing I know of which puts the light back into a man's eyes, and the fire back into his loins, faster than a steak tartare.'

As the basis for this dish, you can use meat cut either from the fillet or rump of the animal, although real experts claim that rump meat is quite superior. Cuts from this part of the animal are generally less tender than sirloin, but the enzyme and red blood corpuscle content is appreciably higher.

Preparing the dish is remarkably easy. The steak is first well spiced with anise, basil, coriander, fennel, sage and garlic and then pounded mercilessly for at least forty five minutes. It doesn't really matter what you use for the pounding, although experts favour wooden camping mallets – the sort normally used for banging tent pegs into the ground. The spicing of the steak is perhaps the most important part of the ritual of preparation. One famous French chef is on record as suggesting that you should use as much spice as you think is necessary and then use as much again.

Type of effect

Raw passion is really for men only. It acts as a sexual stimulant and provides a powerful fillip to the man whose physical capabilities are below par. It has G.O., S.T.A.R.T., P.L.E.A.S.E., M.O.R.E. and S.Q.U.E.A.L. attributes.

Raw Passion is such a powerful male energizer that it is widely used by gigilos and male prostitutes among whom Gigilo's Droop is a recognised occupational hazard.

Speed and length of action

Steak tartare does not begin to have an influence for several hours since the meat and spices must be absorbed into the tissues before any appreciable result can be observed. The steak does, however, retain its potency for two to three days after it has been digested. A man with a pound of raw steak inside him will have ambition and vigor enough to enable him to satisfy most expectations. It is commonly said in Texas that steak tartare, not diamonds, is a girl's best friend.

Warning
A doctor writing in a French journal of international medicine has reported that a woman who gave her husband steak tartare four times a week was admitted to hospital suffering from a fractured pelvis, ruptured uterus and a badly bruised perineum.

Tartar Source

Back in the thirteenth century, the Tartars living in the Mongol Empire had won a justifiable reputation for being rather blood-thirsty. The Siberian Tartars, in particular, were renowed for their savage behaviour and, according to a number of historians, several Siberian Tartar tribes practised cannibalism, supplementing their meagre meat rations by eating their own women-folk. Common soldiers had to make do with the older, stringier females but officers in the Tartar army were entitled to take their pick of the younger girls.

These cannibalistic habits meant, of course, that when it came to taking a bride, Tartar men had to look outside their own community and make raids on distant tribes. Some anthropologists have suggested that the Tartar habit of taking wives from other tribes was evidence of an understanding that intermarriage tends to weaken a closed society. By eating their own women, the Tartars put themselves in a situation where they had no choice but to bring in fresh blood.

Whether Tartar tastes were indeed inspired by a basic understanding of genetics, or whether their habits were fired by more primitive motives such as hunger, the fact remains that the Tartar warriors had to travel to find a spouse.

As the neighbouring tribes became increasingly aware of the threat to their women-folk, so the wife-hungry warriors had to seek further and further afield in search of unattached and unprotected females. They would ride for days, or even weeks, in their quest thundering, apparently tirelessly, across the plains as they sought new tribes and new brides.

Unfortunately, all this travelling meant that by the time they

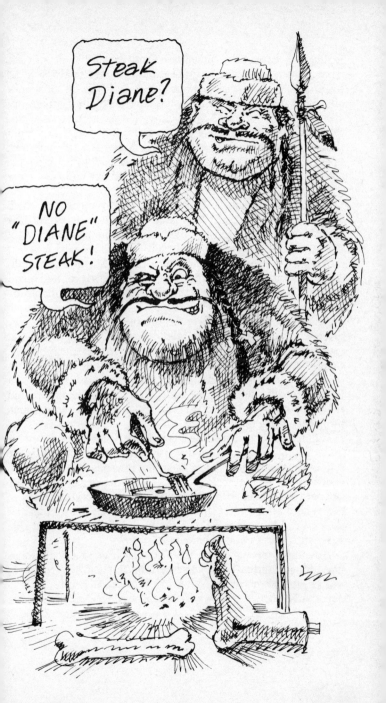

finally did arrive at a village where there were some suitable women, the Tartars were quite exhausted and rarely inclined towards sexual adventure; even if they had been in the mood, after days in the saddle they would have been physically incapable of doing anything about it. Now, that was a grave disadvantage, for the Tartars had long since discovered that if they could seduce their chosen brides before riding back to their own homes, then the aggrieved relatives would not bother to pursue them. Fathers, brothers and suitors would not bother wasting good horse-sweat on soiled goods.

All this meant that the Tartars had to find some way in which they could regain their dissipated strength and revive their sexual enthusiasm. For years they experimented with all sorts of different energy-giving aphrodisiacs. They tried wingless ants embedded in ambergris, they experimented with buttermilk, curry, halibut and imported haggis and they used roasted quail, snail's egg omelettes and peppermint stuffed yams. But nothing seemed to work.

And then, finally, after years of primitive research, they discovered the peculiar properties of raw beef. They found that if they put a well-spiced piece of rump underneath their saddles, then it would be just right for eating by the time they encountered the women of their dreams. As they rode, the friction between saddle, horse's back and Tartar backside would pound the steak into a tender and yet powerful meal – a source of much more than mere nutrition.

When he saw an attractive woman, the Tartar would stop his horse some way off, dismount, rip away the saddle, grab the pulverised steak and swallow it as quickly as possible. Then he'd wait around in the bushes or trees until he began to feel the strength returning to his loins. As soon as everything was in shape he'd lurch out of the undergrowth, grab the woman and ravish her. That done he'd throw her over his horse and ride away with a great whoop of delight.

Anyone observing the antics of couples leaving a steak-house late at night, might recognise certain atavistic tendencies at work. The motor-car has, of course, replaced the horse, and the permissive society makes ravishment less necessary. Still, the modus operandi is the same – as is the stimulant.

KOALA COCOA
Testosterone

Source and preparation

Everyone knows that the quality of human sexuality is influenced by hormones. The sudden surge in the production of specific sex hormones produces the physical changes which take place at puberty and it is the maintenance of those hormone levels which control the masculinity of men and the feminity of women.

It is also known that should those sex hormone levels fall for any reason there will be a diminution in the prominence of sexual characteristics and an accompanying reduction in the capacity to savour to the full the fruits of a physical relationship. It is the level of circulating sex hormones that governs both the quality of the secondary sexual characteristics and an individual's sexual encounters.

Less well understood, perhaps, is the fact that although the shape and size of the female sexual characteristics are governed by oestrogen and progesterone, it is the male hormone testosterone which governs the sexual drive in both men and women. The testosterone level in women is highest during the middle of the reproductive cycle and women are most sexually responsive at that time. If, therefore, one is looking for a hormone with aphrodisiacal qualities the only realistic choice must be testosterone.

The scientists who have worked with testosterone in an attempt to assess its value as an aphrodisiac have, for years, experimented with glandular tissue taken from many different sources. For a while donkey and monkey glands were used. Then tigers' testicles were considered a useful source. But it was not until quite recently that two scientists working in Michigan discovered that the animal which produces a form chemically most akin to human testosterone is the koala bear.

The scientists concerned did a good deal of work on this animal and eventually concluded that the highest concentration of testosterone is found in the undescended testicles of mature bears; which is why, despite violent opposition from a powerful koala bear lobby, there is now a growing army of koala hunters specifically concerned to track down males with undescended testicles. Since the sex of a koala bear is not always easy to determine and since finding the testicles on a koala bear can be a difficult task even when they are descended, it is easy to see why testosterone obtained in this way can fetch extraordinarily high prices.

Fortunately, one testicle usually contains enough testosterone for a single dose. The usual practice is to liquidise the testicle and to prepare a drink with the solution. Because the koala testicle is rather bitter tasting it's advisable to take the extract in a sweet drink. Cocoa is considered particularly suitable since cocoa itself has a mild but subtle aphrodisiacal action.

Type of effect
Testosterone produces a general reaction as a sexual stimulant. Overall the hormone can produce quite dramatic results, particularly in men and women of middle age whose own levels of testosterone are failing.

There is no disinhibiting effect, and no direct effect on orgasmic quality, but testosterone does have G.O., S.T.A.R.T and M.O.R.E. properties.

Speed and length of action
Testosterone usually begins to work within twelve to fourteen days and usually lasts for two to three weeks, though it tends to fade quickly at the end of that time.

Warning
Individuals who have taken koala testosterone forget sometimes that they owe their virility to an aphrodisiac. This can cause problems if the individual concerned forgets to take a refresher dose. Some subjects have been surprised by the speed with which the testosterone effect wears off.

The major's wife
During the three years when I held a commission in the army medical corps, I met very few officers who annoyed me quite as much as Gilbert 'Z'. Gilbert had joined the armed forces while still a student and had been an army veterinary surgeon for nearly twenty years. He always claimed that he'd originally intended to stay in uniform just long enough to see a little of the world but whatever the truth of that may have been, he had eventually settled into a niche which he found comfortable and

entirely satisfying. As a major he had a good reliable income, a considerable amount of authority and a remarkably light work load.

One of Gilbert's more unpleasant traits was an inclination to tell anyone prepared to share a stretch of the bar with him for long enough to listen, that he had only two problems in life. One was his daughter; the other was his wife.

The problem with Sheila 'Z', his daughter, was that although she was still not eighteen years old she had acquired a taste for sexual adventure which had already taken her round the camp's officers and NCOs and had helped her to spread happiness (and non-specific urethritis) through two complete platoons of other ranks.

In complete contrast, his usual complaint about his wife Karen, an exquisite creature some ten years his junior who had married Gilbert when she'd been a junior officer in the army nursing corps, was that her sexual appetites were far less marked than his own.

About six months after I joined the mess, Gilbert came bursting in with the astonishing news that he had just purchased an undescended koala bear testicle from a zoo vet working in Australia. He explained that these organs contain a high proportion of sexually-stimulating hormones and that a single dose, mixed in a drink of cocoa, would agitate the sexual interest of the most torpid partner. His description of what he intended to do to his wife for the two weeks during which the aphrodisiac was guaranteed to work, made several of us feel quite ill. Karen 'Z' was charming, pretty, and as delightful and likeable as her husband was boorish and despicable. Most of the single officers and all the married officers on the camp were in love with her and it was understood quite widely that Karen herself had taken more than a passing fancy to Colonel Tompkins, the camp's extremely popular commanding officer.

'The only snag is that I've got to wait two weeks for it to work,' Gilbert complained with an evil grin.

My colleagues and I agreed there and then that something had to be done to protect the lovely Karen from her unbearable husband's evil plans. We had a fortnight to think of something and we felt sure that we ought to be able to come up with a plan.

In practice, however, it wasn't as easy to find a solution as we'd expected. The only half-decent suggestion – that we somehow arrange for Gilbert's daughter Sheila to drink the adulterated cocoa instead of Karen – had to be abandoned for

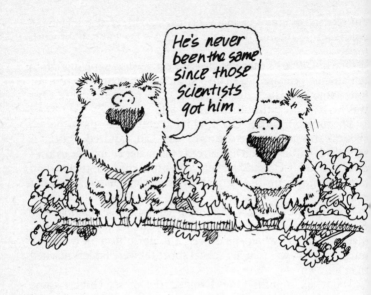

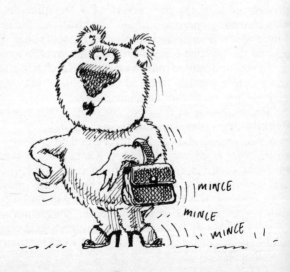

two reasons. First, by the time the suggestion was made it was too late. Secondly, the senior medical officer pointed out that if Sheila spread her non specific urethritis any further, the entire garrison would be inoperative.

For a fortnight we waited, with a growing sense of gloom, for Gilbert to come marching into the bar with a grin on his face and a sordid story to tell. The powerful sense of depression in the mess was only lifted when, on the very day before the testosterone was due to start acting, a subaltern working in the commander's office announced with a smile as broad as a Cheshire cat that Gilbert was being temporarily posted.

'He's leaving tonight and he won't be back for a fortnight,' the young officer announced to loud cheers. 'The Colonel's arranged for him to go on a training course in Iran.'

One or two of the officers in the mess wanted to have a word with the Colonel to find out just how much he'd had to do with Gilbert's temporary posting. But for some inexplicable reason the Colonel could not be found. In fact he was hardly seen at all for a fortnight, and by then the question seemed superfluous.

GLOWMAKER
Green chartreuse

Source and preparation

It has been accepted for centuries that alcohol, by releasing inhibitions and suppressing fears and anxieties, can positively influence sexual behaviour. Alcohol works as an aphrodisiac in two ways. It depresses the restrictive control centres in the brain and thereby allows desires which are normally suppressed to surface. In addition, it causes a general dilatation of the body's superficial blood vessels and thereby produces a generalised skin-glow.

The twin-effect of these two physiological consequences is a mild but appreciable change in the sexual activity of the individual concerned. The depression of normal, restrictive feelings leads to the type of close physical contact in which an accompanying disinhibiting factor can be of great value.

A considerable amount of research has been done in recent years in order to define the optimum dosage of alcohol. Some of the most important work has been done in Paris, where a dedicated Professor has produced powerful evidence to support his contention that the best sexual effect is produced when relatively small doses are employed.

According to the Professor, most women react favourably after drinking between one and one-and-a-half glasses of wine while the majority of men are at their best after two glasses. Men who suffer from premature ejaculation may need three or three-and-a-half, but the vast majority of experimental work has shown that if this sort of dose-range is exceeded the mental capacity might be maintained at a high level but the physical may be reduced.

White wine is generally agreed to be the best general form in which to use alcohol for aphrodisiac purposes. Beers are unsuitable because the heavy fluid intake involved inevitably leads to a need to empty the bladder. Spirits are often unsuitable because of the difficulty in keeping the dosage to a correct level. Red wine is unsuitable for psychological reasons – the colour is subconsciously associated with danger, or with stop-lights.

There is, however, one form of alcohol which seems to have an appreciable advantage over wine; in addition it is particularly suitable for the resistant female. It's green chartreuse: thought to be effective to some small degree because the colour is likely to have a reverse effect on the subconscious from that produced by red wine; but more importantly because chartreuse contains essential oils which slightly irritate the bladder and pelvic region. Many women find this irritation sexually arousing.

Type of effect

When taken in moderation alcohol acts as an excitant on both men and women. Some observers have speculated that alcohol has S.T.A.R.T. qualities, but in fact most professional sexual chemists who have studied alcohol as an aphrodisiac believe that it does not have any such influences. They argue that the initial G.O. effect leads naturally to other things and that these responses are a consequence of the resultant interest in sexual adventure rather than a consequence of any direct physiological change.

The depression of the control centres in the brain also leads to a modest S.I.N. effect during lovemaking and those who are under the influence of alcohol are usually more prone to experiment.

Speed and length of action

Alcohol usually begins to produce results about fifteen minutes after consumption. If food is taken at the same time, however, the rate at which the alcohol is absorbed will be slowed down; this might lead to a more prolonged sexual encounter. Soda water increases the rate at which alcohol is absorbed into the blood stream and concentrates it, but reduces the length of time that its potency will last.

Warning

Alcohol is a very useful general aphrodisiac but is often used inexpertly. Too many people assume that if two glasses are useful then six glasses will be sensational. In truth alcohol is one of the more subtle aphrodisiacs for although it does possess distinct G.O. properties, it will not usually produce dramatic results unless at least one partner is prepared to put a little effort into the proceedings. Those who regard themselves as skilled in the art of seduction consider alcohol to be a substance which must be used with skill and caution.

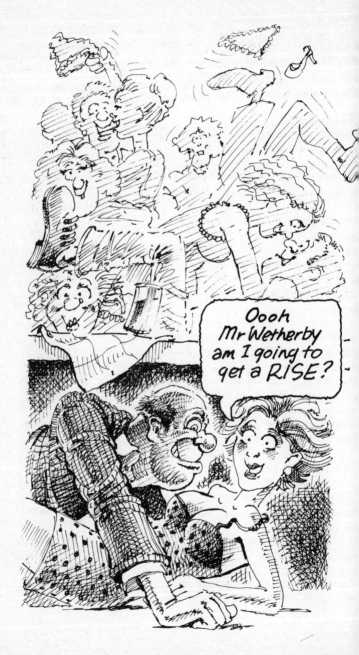

The Christmas Party

The Export Division of Jilks, Kelloware, Harbinger and Nesburton was one of the most imaginative and successful parts of a company which had branches all over the world. It was a Division which frequently managed to negotiate and complete deals which other, less forceful, companies might have considered unlikely. The Division had, for example, at various times in its short history, successfully exported suntan lotion to India, cocktail cabinets to Saudi Arabia, lawn-mowers to Iceland and whisky to Scotland.

Despite its commercial successes, however, the Export Division's Christmas Party had never been an event worth remembering. For weeks before each party the staff would make all the usual preparations. They would hang streamers and balloons from all the light fittings; they would order mince pies and sausage rolls from a local bakery; they would hire drinking glasses and buy enormous supplies of alcohol from a local hostelry and on one occasion they'd even arranged for a disc jockey to bring his records and equipment into the office.

Everything should have gone very well but it never did. Instead of turning into the hoped-for Bacchanalia, the Christmas Party inevitably followed the same dreary pattern. There would be a few speeches and presentations to begin with. Everyone would drink toasts to the chairman, the salesperson of the year, the oldest member of staff and the typist with the longest finger nails. And then they would all get quite hideously and uselessly drunk. In between the speeches and the stupour there was hardly time for a little mischief, let alone a full blown orgy.

From time to time someone would try to do something to improve the quality of the festivities. One year an accounts clerk spiked all the drinks with pure methanol. That simply speeded up the rate at which those attending the party drifted into unconsciousness. Another year, a shorthand typist from the pool brought a handkerchief soaked in LSD, cut it up with the stationery department's power guillotine and handed pieces round. Few of those present could remember what happened but the general concensus of opinion was that it wasn't really worth remembering anyway.

After attending four remarkably unsuccessful parties Henry Taylor, a programmer in the forward planning department of the Division, decided that he would attempt to improve the celebrations in a more scientific way. As the speeches came to an end he made his way through the room carefully topping up everyone's glass with a colourless fluid which he poured from one of a pair of matching silver hip flasks. He concentrated on the younger, prettier, female members of the staff. Every time one of them half emptied her glass he'd top it up. To his delight the plan worked magnificently.

Half-an-hour after the final speech had ended, a buxom typist who worked in the continental accounts division suddenly leapt onto a desk and started to take off her clothes. She was quickly followed by a slender blonde from the filing section and by Mr Harbinger's personal secretary's own personal assistant.

With these three in a state of partial-nudity, the festivities really started to go with a swing. A young salesman who'd just come back from a successful mission in Bulgaria, where he'd sold video recorders to shops in four towns where none of the inhabitants had television sets, managed to persuade a young married woman from the home accounts office to let him undress her with his teeth, while a deputy office manager from the complaints department did much the same sort of thing for a remarkably well built young telephonist. And while all this went on Henry Taylor continued to wander around the room making sure that whenever someone's glass was half empty he was the one to fill it up. Twice he disappeared to replenish his flasks.

Three hours later, the party had developed into a superbly disgraceful affair. Everyone was having a tremendous time. It was the best Christmas Party anyone could remember. Young Henry, content with his work, had abandoned his flasks and settled down with an almost naked photocopier operator and her twin who worked in the duplicating department. As he disappeared under a desk for the third time a colleague, who had lipstick on his collar, face powder on his shirt and a suspender belt round his neck, bent down until his face was no more than six inches from Henry's. 'What did you have in those flasks of yours?' he demanded in a hoarse whisper. 'I must get some of it.'

'It was water,' replied Henry, disappearing underneath a flurry of naked arms and legs. 'Ordinary tap water.'

His colleague didn't believe him but Henry was telling the truth. Most office parties are a disaster because people get too drunk too quickly. By using water to slow down the rate at which the participants became inebriated Henry managed to improve the quality of the party immeasurably. And it really was a *very* good party. No fewer than eleven of the people who attended it never dared show their faces at the office again.

THE WALLBANGER
Dimethyltriptamine

Source and preparation

Dimethyltriptamine is a chemical substance. It has an amphetamine like structure but can produce in those who take it, an hallucinogenic effect which is clinically indistinguishable from that of lysergic acid diethylamide (LSD). In addition to this, dimethyltriptamine dramatically reduces the serotonin levels in the brain.

Although it can be produced in the laboratory by a chemical process which requires only a modest outlay, dimethyltriptamine is more easily available as a naturally occurring triptamine. This substance is found in the resin of a number of trees most of which grow only in South America. Fortunately, the legal restrictions which govern the manufacture and sale of the artificially-produced chemical do not restrict the purification and sale of the naturally occurring triptamine.These triptamine-rich resins are, incidentally, the same substances which have been used by the South American Indians for centuries in the drink *yage* and the snuff *cohoba*.

The traditional South American way of using the resin is to allow it to dry on ordinary parsley and then to make the parsley into a cigarette which can be smoked. Two small drops of undiluted resin provide a dose large enough for most individuals.

Type of effect

The unique virtue of dimethyltriptamine as an aphrodisiac depends partly upon its hallucinogenic value and partly upon the direct effect that the drug has on serotonin levels. In most individuals the hallucinogenic factor produces a feeling of power and megalomania. This initial flood of confidence and self-approval is followed after about ten minutes by such a sense of graciousness, compassion and goodwill towards the world that normally cautious, even selfish, people become outgoing, generous and unusually companionable. It's obvious, then, that dimethyltriptamine tends to be a powerful G.O. and S.T.A.R.T. agent for all who take it.

Those who might normally be shy or withdrawn will become exceptionally, even aggressively, generous. In addition, the lowering of the serotonin levels produces a direct and specific interest in sex, so the overall characteristic of the triptamine is to make those within its power unusually liberal with their sexual favours.

Put simply, dimethyltriptamine can turn the most bashful nun into a raving nymphomaniac.

Speed and length of action

The initial flood of well being lasts for about ten minutes. At the end of this time the individual under the influence of dimethyltriptamine is likely to start forcing sexual favours on the nearest target. The more undemanding and unwilling the target seems to be the more insistant will be the offer.

This combination of goodwill and high-level sexuality peaks for three to five minutes and then slowly subsides. About thirty minutes after the first spasm of well-being, the twin effects of dimethyltriptamine will cease. Since these episodes take place outside the normal range of conscious activity, the individual concerned will have no memory of the incidents which took place under the influence of the drug.

It is important to remember that if the normal dose of dimethyltriptamine is exceeded the drug can be a depressant producing a semi-catatonic state in which the influenced individual has no interest in his or her immediate environment.

Warning

Dimethyltriptamine is known as the 'Wallbanger' because it acts so quickly that immediate sexual activity is largely unavoidable. There is rarely time to seek a physically, legally or socially suitable site. It is important not to expose any individual to the effects of the drug when intercourse would be considered inappropriate, dangerous, embarrassing, or painful.

Rupert Pettigrew's Pursuit of Pleasure

Although I know several people who have used the Wallbanger with a tremendous amount of success, I know of no-one who has succeeded in using this very special aphrodisiac to such good effect as Rupert Pettigrew. I don't think it would be exaggerating too much to say that Pettigrew, who dedicated a good part of his life to using the Wallbanger in the pursuit of pleasure, raised

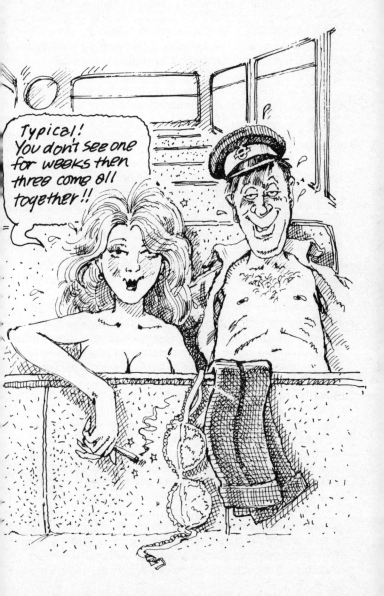

the use of dimethyltriptamine to a minor art form.

Ask Pettigrew where he first got hold of a supply of the Wallbanger and he'll tell you that he can't remember. But he will usually admit (with some pride) that he first used the drug when he was just nineteen years old and back from his first year studying philosophy and economics at Oxford University. At that time he was trying to earn a few pounds working as a temporary postman during the Christmas vacation.

With a pack of specially prepared cigarettes in his anorak pocket, he quickly discovered that delivering letters and cards could be more than just a routine chore. By the time he'd been on the job for four days, he'd got through three packets of Wallbanger cigarettes and a generous clutch of housewives. The groin strain which eventually left him *hors de combat* may well have protected him from more serious injury, since several husbands had begun to harbour suspicions.

Pettigrew found it impossible to settle back into university life after his Christmas holiday job. His studies seemed tame compared to his recent activities; he couldn't concentrate; and more than anything he wanted a chance to perfect his skills with the Wallbanger. So, against the advice of those close to him, Pettigrew left the university and got the first of a series of temporary jobs that would finally earn him a reputation as a drifter and a failure.

Since his main ambition was to experiment with the Wallbanger, Pettigrew took a job as a cab driver thinking that this would provide him with the right sort of opportunities. Opportunities there certainly were, but the problem was that Pettigrew found his conquests too easy. For someone with his skills and imagination, there was no challenge. All he had to do was offer a dimethyltriptamine cigarette and then make sure that he took a route through a fairly secluded part of town. The woman who'd flagged him down and smoked his cigarette would do the rest.

Bored by this, Pettigrew next took a position in a department store, working as a general porter and maintenance man. This time there was more of a challenge. He became adept at walking about on the floor where ladies' dresses were sold and asking customers for a light. Once they'd taken out their matches or lighters it was natural enough to offer them a cigarette. His next move was to ensure that, about ten minutes later, he and the woman were near enough to a changing room to enjoy some privacy. After a month he managed to perfect his style to such a point that he would deliberately select women who were picking out dresses and preparing to try them on. With precise and perfect timing he'd arrange to saunter past the correct changing room at just the right moment. Sadly, he was dismissed when the non-smoking manageress of the lingerie department happened to enter a cubicle where Pettigrew and a customer were enjoying one another. She had thought the sounds emanating from the changing room were those of a plump customer trying on a tight girdle.

After working as a laboratory attendant in a girl's school, a traffic warden in London's West End and a door to door salesman for nuclear fall-out shelters, Pettigrew finally secured a post which he still claims was the pinnacle of his career. He got a job as a bus conductor. By offering cigarettes containing dimethyltriptamine only to those women who had bought tickets for a fairly long trip, by ensuring that he gave those women their cigarettes at a point on the route which meant that ten minutes later they would be between stops, and by keeping the bottom deck filled and the top deck empty, Pettigrew achieved record-breaking successes.

Pettigrew's work on the buses came to a tragic end when the company withdrew their double-decker vehicles and replaced them with single-deckers staffed by a driver-conductor. Not even Pettigrew could succeed against odds like that.

For a few months afterwards Pettigrew worked as a waiter in a large seaside hotel. He missed those happy, challenging days on the buses, however, and became unusually careless. Bad timing meant that he was caught in the hotel dining-room in a position that can only be described as indescribable and shortly afterwards found himself at the local magistrates' court facing a charge of indecent behaviour. His plea that he was inexplicably irresistible to women was accepted after he managed to get himself sexually assaulted by a policewoman – reportedly a heavy smoker – who was due to give evidence in a case of bigamy. As they stood, with many other officers, witnesses and prisoners in an ante-room to the court, Pettigrew offered the hapless girl a cigarette. Ten minutes later, there was chaos in court. A lady magistrate was seen to faint clear away when the rapacious policewoman tore off her uniform and went for Pettigrew's fly; others seemed more inclined to attempt to intervene. At any rate, it was a perfect defence. Pettigrew was given a conditional discharge on the understanding that he take up residence elsewhere. I lost touch with him after that; and I never did find out where he got his supply of Wallbanger.

THE BIG BUZZ
Spanish Fly or cantharis vesicatoria

Source and preparation

Spanish Fly is probably the best-known aphrodisiac. The name itself is rather misleading since the substance did not originally come from Spain and is obtained not from a fly but from a beetle.

Cantharis vesicatoria is a beautiful, shiny insect originally found in the Far East but now fairly common in many parts of Southern Europe. There is, as a matter of record, another member of the same beetle family with similar properties that is found exclusively in Russia. From this cousin an aphrodisiac known as 'Russian Fly' is sometimes concocted.

Spanish Fly has a long history as an aphrodisiac in France. It was, for example, slipped into the soup of Louis XV by Madame de Pompadour, who seemed to spend her life preparing exotic love-potions for her inadequate monarch. Another great French sensualist, the Marquis de Sade, was imprisoned on one occasion for feeding Spanish Fly to an unsuspecting whore.

Obtaining the aphrodisiac is not a difficult process. A number of bettles (say a dozen) should first be anaethetised (experts say that killing the beetles damages their value). They should then be baked until they disintegrate into a fine powder. This powder contains the aphrodisiacal property.

Type of effect

Cantharis vesicatoria has a very general action. It is one of the least subtle and least pleasant aphrodisiacs. Its inclusion in this volume is largely a result of its public reputation rather than its intrinsic value.

The ingredient in Spanish Fly which is aphrodisiacal is a volatile oil which irritates all the body tissues at roughly the same time. It works on the urethra as it is excreted through the urinary tract. The irritation leads the user to imagine that some sort of sexual stimulation must be taking place. Male users have also reported suffering (or enjoying) persistent and abnormally large erections while women have enjoyed (or suffered) massive labial engorgement.

The Spanish Fly is usually classified as having a G.O. effect only, but the stimulation and engorgement of the sexual organs can occasionally have a useful M.O.R.E. quality in both men and women.

Speed and length of action
Spanish Fly does not begin to function until it is excreted through the kidneys and urinary system: a process which takes several hours. Once it has begun, the stimulation usually lasts for six to eight hours, although it has been reported to last for considerably longer.

Warning
Spanish Fly is extremely dangerous. It irritates all the tissues of the body and can cause nephritis, gastroenteritis, cardiac collapse and death. In the nineteen-fifties two young girls in London died when they ate coconut sherbet which had been spiced with the substance. Blending Spanish Fly into cookies or candies can be lethal; indeed after a party in Texas some years ago, seven youths and three girls were taken to hospital with near-lethal malfunctions of their cardiac and digestive systems.

Come fly with me
Many stories are told about the ways in which Spanish Fly has been used to excite sexual interest among those apparently more interested in such activities as the collecting of stamps, the cultivation of roses and the ruling of empires.

Most of the stories concern the attempts made by specific individuals to attract the attention of those not necessarily nearest and certainly not always dearest to them. Disraeli's attempts to coax Queen Victoria out of her widow's weeds with the aid of the famous Fly and Pasteur's use of the drug to excite and interest the young Marie Curie are rumoured to be just two examples of the ways in which this particular aphrodisiac has been used.

One of the most dramatic and extraordinary uses of the drug did not, however, involve just two individuals, but an entire community. It happened in a small Swedish town just south of Stockholm – a town which, for legal reasons, still cannot be named. Litigation started as a result of the Fly's use is still unresolved.

The story begins with a local druggist, whom I shall refer to as Mr Y. He owned and ran a small general pharmacy in which he sold the usual variety of goods. He had a pharmacist's licence, he

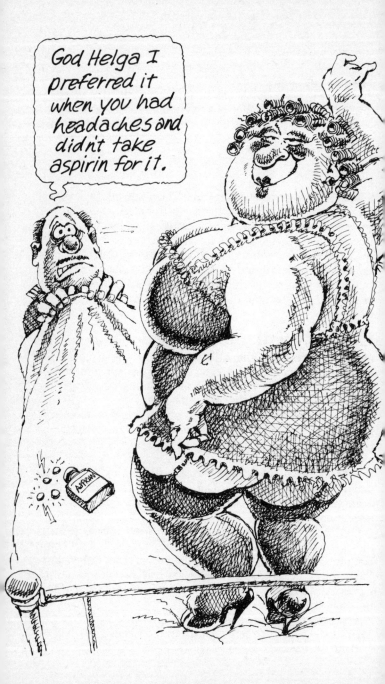

78

dispensed prescriptions, and conducted a small trade in such items as hot water bottles, contraceptives and toothbrushes. Most of his business involved non-prescription medicines: cough linctus, indigestion mixtures and tonics. It was this part of Mr Y's business which enabled him to have such an influence on his fellow citizens and eventually led to one of the most extraordinary scandals in modern Swedish history.

Many commentators have tried to decide precisely what led the druggist to believe that the declining birth-rate in Sweden was threatening his country's future and putting the success of his own business at risk. Suggestions were made that his motive was personal (i.e. sexual) but I don't think anyone ever produced evidence to support that theory. Mr Y may well have taken advantage of the change in sexual behaviour which occurred locally as a result of his activities, but I think it is unfair to suggest that his motives were as selfish as that. It is probably true that the fall in demand for nappies, and other baby products had begun to affect his business dramatically. Whatever the reason may have been, however, the simple fact is that Mr Y decided that he had to do something to reverse the trend.

His solution was remarkably simple. He bought a huge supply of cantharis vesicatoria from a Dutch wholesaler. Then, having taken delivery of the consignment, he proceeded, carefully and systematically, to lace every single patent medicine that he sold. The bottles of cough medicine, the stomach calmative, the aspirin tablets, and the de-worming medicines were all given a dash of cantharis. They were turned from simple, harmless home-medicines into sexually stimulating time bombs.

Since he was a qualified chemist and had, or so it appears, no desire to harm any of his customers, he was careful to ensure that the dose of cantharis he used was so small that it would not do any damage. Despite which it was more than enough to stimulate the sexual appetites of his customers – and they constituted most of the township's population.

The results were just as Mr Y had hoped. Despite the fact that the sales of contraceptives rocketed, the birth rate rose steadily. There were a few divorces and a few hurried marriages too, but on the whole the social fabric of the town was not unduly disturbed.

The plan may well have gone quite unnoticed if it had not been for the fact that one of his customers decided to take an overdose of aspirin tablets. Sadly, for Mr Y she died not of aspirin poisoning but from a superfluity of cantharis. At the inquest which followed her death the pathologist announced to an astonished courtroom that the tablets that had caused the woman's death had been laced with Spanish Fly.

The uproar was tremendous. And although a number of citizens spoke on behalf of the pharmacist, others were less than pleased to hear that they had been influenced in such an underhand way. Days after the inquest, Mr Y found himself besieged by lawyers bearing writs from parents who wanted him to pay maintainance for their children, from girls who wanted him to pay for their abortions and from men who wanted compensation for their loss of freedom. The denouement of this story is somewhat unclear. Mr Y was arraigned and a date set for his trial. Some days before he was due to appear in court, he managed to escape from prison, cross the border and effectively disappear – almost certainly with the aid of forged papers and a fake passport. It's obvious that he couldn't have done this without help: and pretty influential help at that. So it would seem that not all his customers were angry or disappointed!

DOUBLES BAR
Chocolate

Source and preparation

Montezuma, the Aztec King, collected wives the way other men collect hotel towels or bookmatches. By the time he'd begun to settle into a life of more or less 'normal' domesticity, he'd acquired a harem of seven-hundred beauties. Keeping that number of women happy in bed would pose a few problems for most men, but Montezuma obtained the necessary stamina and sexual strength by drinking huge quantities of a special beverage. He even had a little strength left over to deal with a few affairs on the side.

The basic ingredient of the King's own brew was chocolate, something traditionally used by the Aztecs in ceremonies that honoured Xochiquetzal, their unique and generous Goddess of Love. To remain capable of satisfying those seven-hundred members of the Royal Household the good King got through an average of fifty cups of chocolate a day.

Chocolate was introduced into Spain in the early seventeenth century. Its use spread throughout Europe as its value as an aphrodisiac became apparent: first by the Spanish themselves, then by the French and finally by the Italians. By the mid eighteenth century the potency of chocolate as an aphrodisiac had been called into question; and by the nineteenth it was thought of as a token of affection rather than as a love-making aid. Indeed, it was not until researchers in New York discovered that chocolate contains a chemical called phenylethylamine, which has a powerful stimulatory effect on the emotional responses of those who take it, that the real value of chocolate was re-established.

If this recent research is to be believed, then the Aztecs really knew what they were doing. Chocolate, it seems, stimulates the emotions and helps provide consumers with the physical capacity to enjoy their new found aspirations.

Chocolate is, of course, available in very many different forms but it is important to remember that in order to obtain the fullest physical and mental benefit from this aphrodisiac, fairly large quantities need to be taken. Although boxes of chocolate with soft centres are a traditional romantic gift, the fact is that there's not enough chocolate in a one pound box of soft centres to do more than titillate the sexual palate.Four or five cups of drinking chocolate or two or three half pound slabs are needed if any useful result is to be obtained.

Type of effect
Chocolate has two quite separate qualities. Its effect on the frontal lobes of the brain makes it an excitant for both males and females. Through the same neurological pathways, slightly larger quantities of chocolate have S.T.A.R.T. properties. A single half-pound slab of solid chocolate taken three times a day will work wonders. Twice that quantity will invariably produce quite dramatic results. Very large quantities of chocolate will have an effect on the quality of orgasm.

Speed and length of action
A world-famous chef is reported to have claimed that chocolate usually begins to produce a noticeable change in sexual attitudes within three hours of consumption. Others observers however, have suggested that potency will reach a peak some four to four and half hours later, last for between two and three hours, and then slowly wear off during the following six to eight hours.

Warning
There are two significant problems with this particular type of aphrodisiac. First, many individuals are unable to tolerate the quantity of chocolate which must be consumed. Secondly, since the calorie value of chocolate is high, regular consumption can lead to a considerable weight problem. By the time he celebrated his forty-fifth birthday (when he took an extra forty-five wives) Montezuma was so obese that he was unable to move from his bed. In order to overcome the problems associated with the King's exceptional girth, his wives were lowered into position by a slave-operated hoist.

Marcia, the reluctant virgin
By the age of eighteen, Marcia Barmouth had developed into an astonishingly beautiful young woman. She had a perfect complexion, long, silky brown hair, an exquisite figure and a pair of ever-twinkling eyes. Wherever she went, she attracted men as surely as a flower in the pollen season will attract bees. But although she was flattered by the attention she received, and

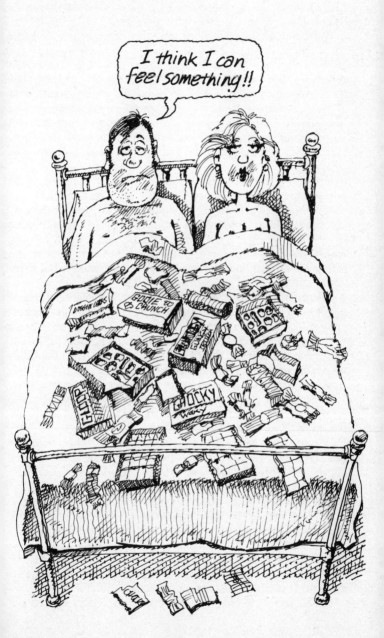

although she desperately wanted to enjoy the company of the men she met, young Marcia had a problem that she was quite unable to overcome: she was extremely shy.

Even though she had been out with half-a-dozen different men she still hadn't been kissed. She certainly hadn't ever enjoyed any of the sensual thrills that her friends had been reporting. Whenever a man persuaded her to let him escort her for the evening, she would go out with every intention of allowing herself to enjoy – even encourage – his advances. She desperately wanted to be kissed. She desperately wanted to feel a loving man's strong hands on her firm young body . . . She'd read plenty of romantic novels and she knew what it ought to be like.

Yet somehow it never worked out quite like that. They would enjoy dinner together, or perhaps share a pleasant evening at the theatre or cinema. Then, inexplicably, Marcia's good intentions and brave ambitions would be submerged by an overwhelming wave of insecurity and self-consciousness. Gently but firmly she would resist any advances. She knew that later, back in the safety of her own bed, she would regret her timidity, but there wasn't anything that she could do about it.

Eventually, in desperation, Marcia confessed all this to one of her dearest and closest friends. She explained that she desperately wanted to live a little more dangerously. She was shy and timid but deep inside there burned the unquenchable passion of a true romantic in search of physical adventure, spiritual fulfilment and an uncertain emotional destiny.

Marcia's friend listened with sympathy and compassion. 'What you need,' she pointed out, 'is an aphrodisiac you can use on yourself. Something to release your shackles and leave you free to fly.'

When, after some thought, Marcia agreed that that was exactly what she needed her friend suggested that she try chocolate. 'You must eat several large bars of it every day,' she warned, 'but then you'll soon find yourself taking advantage of all the offers you're getting.'

As Marcia's friend had forecast, what followed was quite dramatic. On her first date, after starting the chocolate regime, Marcia permitted a kiss. On her second date she allowed a boy to unfasten her blouse. On her third date she took the initiative herself. And on the morning after her fourth date she made an appointment with the local family planning clinic.

For three months Marcia's life was idyllic. She followed her new sexual diet with great vigour and enthusiasm. She bought chocolate bars by the boxful and consumed them at an astonishing rate. She spent her lunch hours buying up bars of chocolate and her evenings eating them. She downed vast quantities of milk chocolate, plain chocolate, cooking chocolate, Swiss chocolate and powdered drinking chocolate.

All Marcia's dreams and fantasies had become reality. She enjoyed the romantic and sexual attentions of half a dozen skilled, eager lovers. She obtained great pleasure from these relationships and slowly began to forget how shyness and timidity had once been such inhibiting forces in her life.

And then, slowly and quite inexplicably, things began to go wrong. One by one, the men she'd been seeing stopped calling for her. Where, once, there had been an unending series of suitors at the door and on the telephone, there were now none. Marcia had replaced opportunity without inclination for inclination without opportunity.

Sadly she confessed all this to her friend, the kind companion who had taught her the value of chocolate.

'Why don't I seem to attract men any more?' she asked. 'I don't even get wolf-whistles from lorry drivers now.'

'Have you looked at yourself lately?' her friend asked, perhaps a little unkindly. 'Your skin is greasy, your face is covered in spots and you must be fifty pounds overweight.' Poor Marcia had learned exactly what people mean when they talk about the bitter-sweet taste of chocolate.

An unhappy ending? No, not really. Marcia gave up chocolate and went on a crash diet. Within a month or two her skin had cleared, the fat had fallen away and she had regained the beautiful face and figure that had attracted her eager lovers. The lack of chocolate no longer mattered: she had overcome the paralysing shyness that, at one time, had saddened her life. Once embarked on a life of sensual pleasure, she didn't need the aphrodisiac's artificial aid . . . though I gather that she still enjoys the occasional slice of chocolate-layered gateau.

PARTY LINE
Datura, the jimson weed

Source and preparation

There are said to be more than twenty species of datura which have hallucinogenic properties. However, only two kinds of datura are native to the western hemisphere: datura stamonium and datura inoxia. The second of these has such a powerful hallucinogenic effect that preparations made from it have reportedly been used to help lure young girls into prostitution. It is, therefore, the first plant, datura stramonium, or thorn apple as it is known in Europe, which has the most practical worth as an aphrodisiac.

The active ingredients of datura stramonium which give it its erotic value include hyoscine and scopolamine – scoplamine being, of course, the mind-bending drug widely used by interrogators.

Since the plant can be eaten in its raw state it is sometimes served up in salads (datura acquired the name jimson weed after it was accidentally added to salads given to soldiers billeted in Jamestown, Virginia). It is, however, more common to isolate the aphrodisiac ingredient by drying the leaves of the plant, putting a teaspoonful onto a plate, igniting the residue with a match (a petrol or gas lighter will damage the quality of the fumes) and then inhaling the smoke. Thorn apple cigarettes can also be prepared.

Type of effect

Datura has several unique qualities. Since it contains scopolamine it tends to have a most remarkable disinhibiting trait. Those who have used it regularly claim that it enables users to enjoy their most erotic fantasies without fear since it breaks down all existing social and cultural barriers.

Because of its value as an aid to the enjoyment of sexual fantasies, datura is commonly employed by onanists; but its most remarkable value perhaps was that described by Dr Joseph Huttle, adviser to an American sociological institute, in a monograph published in 1971. Dr Huttle reported that a growing number of travelling businessmen have taken to using the datura plant to help them satisfy their wives while they themselves are abroad. The husband and the wife, connected only by telephone, ignite their datura at the same time and by this means are able to enjoy a mutual fantasy.

Speed and length of action
Datura works almost instantaneously on those who inhale the smoke and lasts for some thirty or forty minutes. One of the most remarkable things about it is that once the experience ends, those who have used the drug are sometimes unable to remember anything that has happened.

Warning
Many herbalists use thorn apple smoke as a cure for asthma. This practice tends to bring unexpected joy to many patients and unexpected profit to many herbalists. Those who use datura as a telephone aid should be aware that several cases of bell ringer's fist have been recorded and associated with this aphrodisiac.

Togetherness
Daphne Redworth first heard about the thorn apple when she, Mary Gingham, Ellen Dabchick and Nora Galloway were round at Polly Walker's for an evening meeting of the St Dunstan's sewing circle. The five of them met once a week in one another's homes. Theoretically, they met to discuss new sewing patterns and compare handiwork, but since none of them was particularly interested in sewing, the business part of their meetings rarely took up much more than five minutes or so. They usually spent the remainder of the evening playing poker, telling raunchy stories and emptying gin bottles.

Polly Walker's husband was a travelling representative who spent a lot of time away from home and was currently in the middle of a two week trip to Spain. Sometimes when her husband was away Polly would encourage her friends to stay as long as they could. Their meetings often went on until one or even two in the morning.

That evening, however, Daphne sensed that something was different. Polly kept looking at her watch, emptying the ash trays and fiddling with the cushions. By half past ten she was sitting on the edge of her chair; the butts from fifteen or so cigarettes were crushed in the ashtray in front of her. Four times in the space of ten minutes she'd emptied her gin glass and four

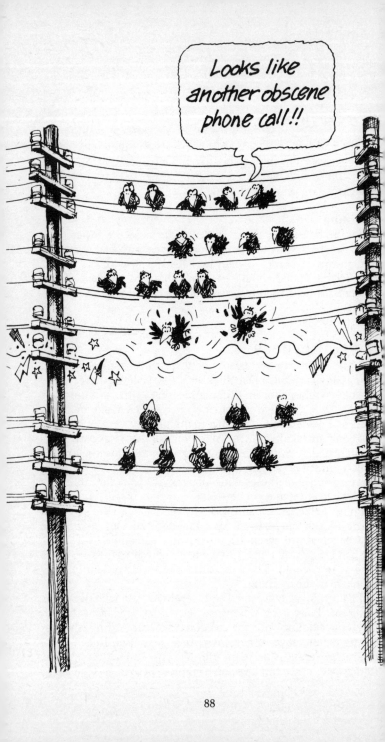

times Nora Galloway had filled it up again for her.

'Do you want us to go?' asked Daphne as Polly shook her watch for the fourth time in a minute.

'Oh, must you?' said Polly, jumping up, emptying her glass again and stubbing out another cigarette. 'What a pity! It's so early. Still we'll be seeing one another next week. Don't worry about the washing up.'

'You've got something planned for tonight, haven't you?' said Ellen Dabchick, winking so outrageously that half a false eyelash came loose. She, Mary, Daphne and Nora hadn't moved an inch. It was clear that they had no intention of moving. So poor Polly really didn't have any option but to tell all. She explained (at first with some diffidence) how she and her husband had recently discovered that even if they were several thousand miles apart they could enjoy a successful sexual relationship simply by talking to one another on the telephone while inhaling smoke from burning thorn apple. She'd been browsing through an old book on herbal remedies – part of a job-lot she'd bought at a St Dunstan's bring-and-buy sale – when she'd come across the reference to thorn apple and its interesting side-effects. She and her husband had tried it out and discovered that it worked; and now it had become an indispensable part of their forced separations.

Her friends were sceptical at first; then curious; then downright eager. Consequently, when the telephone rang at eleven that evening the five of them were huddled around it with a tablespoonful of thorn apple sitting on a plate between them and a box of matches at the ready. It was a real ring of confidants.

Descriptions of what followed vary according to which member of the sewing circle you listen to, but each lady agreed afterwards that it would all have been quite impossible if Polly's husband had not thoughtfully arranged for one of those telephone loudspeaker attachments to be fitted to his home 'phone. The device may have been intended to free Polly's hands but it also made it possible for Mary, Nora, Daphne and Ellen to listen to her conversation with Harry.

Nora still insists that Harry Walker must have heard Mary Gingham giggling and Mary claims that Harry must have heard Nora's only very slightly muffled squeals of delight. But whether Harry guessed that his wife had visitors that evening no one ever really knew for sure. And no one felt like telling him that his own groans of delight had been shared five ways.

Each of Polly's visitors claims to be enjoying a fuller life thanks to thorn apple: possibly because they all have husbands who travel a lot. Daphne told me that she and her husband first tried out the thorn apple when they were parted by a Frankfurt Industrial Fair. It was an inauspicious start. It seems that the operator, who was eavesdropping, reached her own climax before they did and became so excited that she broke the connection. Even so, they've continued to use the aphrodisiac when circumstance parts them; and, like all Polly's friends, agree that it gives a new dimension to the notion that absence makes the heart grow fonder.

ATTITUDE ADJUSTMENT APPLIANCES

Repertoire

Clothes are an obvious sexual device. Black stockings, high-heeled shoes, uplift bras, bikini panties, garter-belts, leather trousers, skin-tight sweaters, low-cut dresses, G-strings, tight jeans, flimsy see-through nighties – these are just some of the most commonly-employed and best-known attitude adjustment appliances. By carefully selecting what we choose to wear, it is possible to make clear our sexual availability, our preferences and our prejudices. It is always worth remembering though, that what an individual wears in public may vary considerably from what is worn for the special delight of a favoured lover. A woman clad in a simple black dress which suggests that she is thoughtful, serious and quite proper may wear beneath it a set of lacy, revealing black lingerie which demonstrates to those allowed beyond what's on view that she is far more daring, sexually sophisticated and adventurous than they might have imagined.

Cosmetics, too, have been used for centuries by those wanting to make themselves more alluring. Lipstick, eyeshadow, perfume, bath-oil, hair-colourant, rouge, eyeliner, nail-varnish, face-powder – the list goes on and on. Few women allow themselves to be seen without their make-up and the sexual value of these products can be easily judged by the way in which they are marketed. Perfumes are advertised as irresistible to men, while bath oils are promoted with a hint of illicit sexual adventure to come. Lipsticks are sold in a blatantly suggestive way with photographs of girls with moist, half-open lips poised above the blood red cylinders of colour. There is rarely any doubt in the mind of the manufacturer, or the consumer, that what is being retailed is much, much more than could be sold in a tube or a bottle.

Skin decorations of slightly different kinds have become increasingly popular in recent years. Many men and women are attracted by tattoos and a growing number of girls have small, delicate pictures permanently engraved on their breasts. Even more surprising, perhaps, is the fact that a number of young girls are today having their nipples pierced and threaded with small rings and chains. This practice was common in England at the start of the nineteenth century, but it is now popular throughout the world. Incidentally, in ancient Egypt it was common for a man to have miniature bells surgically attached to the penis just below the glans. Some popular modern songs celebrate this remarkable tradition.

Aids designed to directly influence the length and strength of the orgasmic experience are available in many different forms. There are penile rings to help maintain the erection, 'french ticklers' to help stimulate the clitoris, mechanical vibrators to help augment standard stimulatory techniques, or to help in the practice of automanipulation, and a whole range of other gadgets and devices.

Finally, books and magazines which contain photographs and stories of a stimulating nature are very easily available today. Some of the more traditional publications use professional models and writers and simply offer visual food for the satisfaction of the cerebral appetites. There are, however, a growing number of publications which encourage readers to participate by producing photographs and stories of their own. These demonstrate a growing interest in self-help.

Type of effect

This usually depends upon the sexual aims and erotic ambitions of those involved. (Some devices may be particularly fitting for lonely individuals, but the majority of the appliances discussed in this section are designed for two or more participants.)

Low cut dresses, tightly cut jeans and the cruder types of cosmetic are designed to have a non specific G.O. effect. Other appliances, such as penile rings and decorated condoms are intended for use as P.L.E.A.S.E., M.O.R.E. and S.Q.U.E.A.L. devices.

Speed and length of action

This quality depends largely upon the inherent sexual capacities of the individuals using them. With the exception of devices designed to boost performance, most attitude adjustment appliances are designed to release hidden desires. They are excitants which depend for their effectiveness on unrealised sexual aspirations.

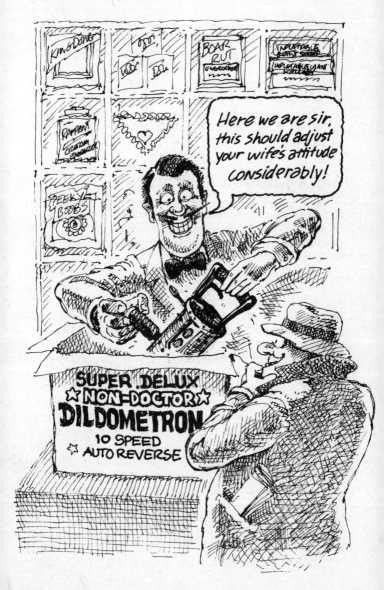

Warning

Attitude adjustment appliances which are designed and used for a specific purpose produce little in the way of problems. A woman who has deliberately and provocatively dressed in black stockings and garter-belt is unlikely to be surprised or disappointed by the response she elicits from her lover.

On the other hand, appliances which are used without any specific target in sight can produce all sorts of problems. Those who use them may find themselves embarrassed if they provoke unwelcome reactions. Conversely, those who respond to the allure of a member of the opposite sex who has unconsciously employed attitude adjustment appliances which enhance his or her sexual attraction, may be disappointed when encountering an angry rebuff.

Miss Jackson's plumage

When the fourteen men working in the offices of Whychberry and Whychberry, Chartered Accountants, heard that a young woman was going to join them as a junior assistant they held a meeting to discuss what was, for them, an event as momentous as the invention of the calculator.

Some of the older members of the firm were apprehensive at first. They feared that their reputation as respectable, if slightly well-starched, members of an honourable profession would be damaged by the arrival of a young woman. But Mr Whychberry, the firm's bachelor chairman, was far more enthusiastic. He pointed out that having a woman around the place would add to the firm's appeal – it would appear less stuffy, perhaps – and in the long run would be good for business. This last argument was, of course, a most powerful one and eventually the men agreed to welcome the newcomer as an equal. Moreover, they determined to show her that although they had no previous experience of women colleagues, they were quite capable of moving with the times and resolved to avoid any kind of discrimination or harassment. What, in their innocence, they had not realised is that harassment (and sexual harassment in particular) can take many forms. The new assistant at Whychberry's hadn't been there for more than a few hours before it became clear that if anyone was going to do any harassing it wasn't going to be the male members of the company but the newcomer.

Although she was barely out of her teens, April Jackson was

xtremely adept at making the best of her natural talents: and ney were many. Between her neck and her waist her contours ook the longest possible way round.

For her first morning at the office she wore a diaphanous louse that would have revealed a good extent of cleavage even if he'd fastened all the buttons. The sight was guaranteed to tillate even the most jaded palate. Her buttock-hugging skirt as short enough to reveal to anyone remotely interested in nding out that she wore stockings and suspenders. Miss ackson's arrival at the staid offices of Whychberry in a cloud of rench perfume was the most memorable event in the firm's istory since the legendary fire of 1904.

As the weeks went by it became more and more apparent that Miss Jackson's disruptive influence was unlikely to wane. Using rare natural skill, she succeeded in disturbing her fellow mployees in a subtle and yet remarkably efficient way. When he wore a blouse it was always low-cut. When she wore a dress it as always skin-tight. If she wore trousers they were always gure-hugging.

Nor was the harassment confined to her choice of clothes. She eemed to have a flair for creating the greatest amount of havoc the most simple and seemingly inoffensive way. If she had to end over to pick anything up, she always bent from the waist so aat her bottom was provocatively elevated. If she happened to e wearing a dress or blouse with a particularly low neck she eemed to take every opportunity to lean forward when chatting a colleague. Mature men who thought they had lost the talent or eroticism would become faint with excitement whenever Miss Jackson borrowed a pencil or a paperclip. She taunted, she irted and she teased.

Not surprisingly this technique took its toll. The company's eputation fell. Accounts were delayed. Auditing errors were ommonplace. For the first time in its history, Whychberry was areatened by financial problems. Once a firm of chartered ccountants loses its good reputation it quickly loses its clients. Money is a serious business and people expect their accounts to e handled with care, caution and discretion.

Three months after Miss Jackson's arrival, Mr Whychberry as forced to call a meeting of his thirteen colleagues to ask for neir advice and help. For several hours they discussed this most nusual of problems, eventually agreeing that they could not ossibly fire her as unsuitable, since her work was faultless and ny dismissal would be likely to attract adverse comment. There

was, they all agreed at last, only one possible answer to thei
problem.

And so, two months later, a delighted Miss Jackson retire
from office work and became Mrs Wychberry. Those wh
assumed that the chairman's new wife would spend her day
dressed in nothing more substantial than two ounces of silk an
dedicate her life to teasing the milkman, the postman and th
window-cleaner would have been surprised to learn that Mr
Wychberry became, in fact, the very model of propriety. Sh
dressed in sensible jumpers and skirts and favoured a heavy
quilted dressing gown when obliged to answer the door to
tradesman early in the morning. The plumage she had em
ployed as a girl with ambitions had been discarded when it ha
served its purpose. Mark you, the equipment might have bee
abandoned, but the sensuality it represented remained. M
Wychberry, after his marriage, took to arriving at the office a
ten-thirty and never leaving later than four p.m. Lon
weekends became a part of his routine; and his colleagues had t
agree that although he had developed an irritating tendency t
fall asleep in meetings, he'd never seemed happier.